D1636838

RETURN TO SENDER

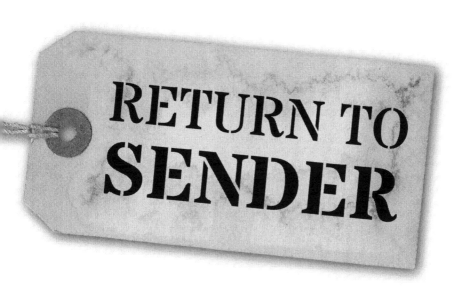

RETURN TO SENDER

A Collection of
Medical Advocacy Stories
Through the Eyes of a Nurse

ANDREA S. KOHN, RN CRNP

Dedication

This book is dedicated to my Sender for giving me the parents and extended family He gave me. As my oldest son frequently says, "We won the lottery of life." This is truly how I feel, and I thank my parents for raising me to be grateful, believe in myself, be respectful of others, and never let anyone "steal my joy." My mother was a nurse who mentored me by showing me how to care for family, neighbors, and patients in a way that honored our profession. She cared for anyone in the family who needed help. She brought both of her parents home to our house while she cared for their every need and never vented frustration in their final season of life. She demonstrated quality of life and what "no regrets" truly looks like until her last day on this Earth.

I am also grateful to my grandparents, the city Jews from Philly and the country Christians from the hills of Pennsylvania, for showing unity through love and teaching me that two different religions can blend together and love unconditionally with God at the helm.

I am grateful to my husband, Steve, for being my rock and being open to a crazy life that we have woven together with many different threads: raising three sons lovingly, of supporting our parents in good times and bad, but most of all, of joining me in our business of providing services primarily to the elderly in need. Steve has been teachable. He has become a pro at engaging our clients, showing concern, and truly caring about them and their circumstances. Our business has been blessed, and we are grateful to each family that has entrusted us to care for their loved one. We have felt privileged to have this role and have learned vastly more through our experiences than any textbook could convey.

I am grateful to my village of extended family: four zany brothers, their wives and their children, and now their children. Each brother showed love and compassion in a different way but always provided comedic relief in our family, even when humor seemed out of reach. Each grandchild and great-grandchild brought joy to our parents' hearts and enriched their lives with their love on every visit to their home. I am thankful for cousins in Florida, Pennsylvania (BC and SBC), and New Jersey. I am thankful for our settlement in Lanse and Ridgway and for our forefathers in Sweden and the Ukraine. I am thankful for my friends that are my chosen family: my Cedarbrook family, my school days family, "the pack," and my neighborhood family. I am thankful for all the mentors in my life and for all the physicians that effected change in my life and in my loved ones' lives, personally as well as professionally. Much gratitude to Dr. Urquhart, Dr. Soliman, Dr. Goyal, Dr. Olin, Dr. Nagel, Dr. Wells, Dr. Norvell, Dr. Pushkas, Dr. Schiffman, Dr. Schneider, Dr. Gilbert, and Dr. Schor. I am thankful for every caregiver that I have ever had the pleasure to work beside; you have blessed my life.

Much gratitude to Terry RN, Amy RN, Mary and Alan, Lisa and Bill, Bonnie and Barry, Cathy and Bob, Kelli and John, Kathy, Kate, and Tighe for support that is unmatched and for being there for us no matter what! I owe you all! Special mention to Clara, Margo, Lia, and Nellie for making Mom's extra chapters even happen and for loving on her like you did.

Thank you to my sons for your unconditional love and for allowing me to be your mother and for forgiving me for any bad parenting decisions that I made. You are still helping me to grow up and be a better person. I wish for you and your children the blessings and life that I have been given and then some. Always be "humble and kind" and pass on what you have been given.

Always laugh, always learn, and always love. Always channel our Angel Mom-mom and what she taught us!

With a grateful heart,

Andrea

"Working hard for something we don't care about is called stress. Working hard for something we love is called passion."

– Simon Sinek

Contents

· Chapter 1 ·

Only a Miracle

"I can choose how I'm going to regard unfortunate circumstances in my life—whether I will see them as curses or opportunities . . . I can choose my words, and the tone of voice in which I speak to others. And most of all I can choose my thoughts."

—Elizabeth Gilbert

"Only a miracle will save him . . ." Those words, spoken to us by my father's doctor, resonated in my mind over and over. When confronted with a statement like this from an experienced physician, I knew the situation was dire.

"Miracles" are not routinely discussed as a part of one's medical care. I remember grasping the sides of my head, grabbing the closest seat, putting my head down, and being flooded with a typhoon of emotions as I began the "What now?" process. My father, who had an amazing sense of humor, was quick witted, and very mild mannered; who represented strength, character, integrity, and intelligence; who was a math whiz and could do any calculation in his brain or tell you within thirty seconds the day of the week for any past date, was an amazing, kind father who loved his family well and never met a stranger. But now his life was suddenly hanging in the balance, and here we were embarking upon an unplanned, frightening journey with no road map. Hope is the one emotion we cling to in situations of high stress, so we did just that.

The day began like any other day in early 1988. I took the Metro to work at George Washington University Hospital to review hospital records for billing analysis purposes, which was my job at the time. I received a call in the late morning at work from my mother telling me that my father was in a local hospital with a bleeding peptic ulcer, his second such admission for this. I asked if she thought it was urgent for me to get there, and she said she didn't think so. Since my mother had been a nurse herself for over thirty-seven years, I trusted her judgement. She felt the situation was under control, and the doctors felt confident that they could stop the bleeding quickly. Although I was also a nurse, I was still rather "green." Despite what my mom said, my role as a daughter kicked in, and I rushed to the hospital as a support for both my parents. After all, my mother was alone in the role of overseeing all the medical decisions for my father, with the help of the doctors on the case, and weighing any and all options with very little time to contemplate. My four brothers were not in the medical field and also relied heavily on our mother for medical guidance.

Day one seemed like everything would be OK as the doctors seemed to have it under control. They were trying to get the bleeding stopped, and they had several options to try before they opted to do surgery. As the day progressed, it seemed that the bleeding slowed down a bit, but he was not completely responding to the procedures that they were attempting. In the late afternoon, we were called into a conference room where they told us that while Dad was "stable," he was continuing to slowly bleed from his stomach ulcer, and they would need to go in and do surgery to stop the bleeding. They told us they would monitor him through the night and prepare him for surgery; IVs, medication, and lab tests were all being done.

They scheduled for the next day, a subtotal gastrectomy, a surgery to remove part of my father's stomach. Dad, who was sixty-four years old at the time, had been diagnosed with adult-onset juvenile diabetes at the age of thirty-seven and was immediately put on insulin, had a blood disorder known as polycythemia vera (viscous blood), and had a prosthetic eye due to diphtheria as a child. Leading up to this admission, my father received excellent routine medical care by a primary care physician who also specialized in hematology/oncology. He had an endocrinologist who was on top of his diabetes, and his polycythemia vera was stable. Dad was a compliant patient, barring the occasional slice of cake he would sneak behind my mother's back.

Proper management of chronic disease processes, such as type 1 diabetes, is pivotal for positive outcomes. As a registered nurse, my mother took meticulous care of her primary patient, my father. She was a bit of a drill sergeant who we knew had served him well as she was fastidious about his diabetic diet. She knew that by adhering to a strict diabetic diet and managing his blood sugars within a safe range, she would ultimately enhance his quality of life and minimize the target organ damage—organs targeted by the disease—that accumulates with blood sugars that are not properly maintained. This requires routine finger pricks that then guide how much insulin one is to take, as the problem with type 1 diabetes is that individuals do not produce enough insulin on their own. If blood sugars are not monitored carefully, target organ damage to the heart, blood vessels, nerves, eyes, and kidneys occurs over time, leading to long-term irreversible damage. Mom happily assumed this role as Dad's patient advocate early on in their marriage. While Dad was appreciative of her role, he was not always pleased when told that he could not have that piece of pecan pie or birthday cake based on the number of carbohydrates. It was a family joke that all sweets had to be hidden from Dad, although he often snuck into the next room to graze on a piece of cake, forgetting to see if he left icing on his cheek, a dead giveaway!

By now, we had contacted our family members and closest friends to let them know that our dear dad was in trouble and in the hospital. We activated our village community that swung right into action and began dropping food off for us, helping with pets at home, and just supporting us during a time when we most needed it. These folks just seemed to know what we needed and when, even if it was just to sit with us in the hospital for an hour and be a listening ear.

On day two the surgery appeared to be successful, and my father was admitted to a post-surgical unit of the hospital where things seemed to be fine. After a long day of keeping him company at the bedside, we kissed him goodnight and told him we would see him in the morning. We went home and went to bed. A phone call at 3 a.m. awakened me. My father had taken a turn for the worse and was now in the Intensive Care Unit (ICU), so we needed to go to him immediately. I drove to my mom's house and picked her up.

We arrived at the hospital where we were given the dire news of "only a miracle will save him." My father had begun to bleed from his incision site and multiple sites internally due to a condition called Disseminated Intravascular Coagulation (DIC), which the National Institutes of Health defines as, "a rare but serious condition that causes abnormal blood clotting throughout the body's blood vessels . . . and makes the body's normal blood clotting process become overactive." This is a very rare condition, with fewer than

20,000 cases per year in the US. Approximately 50 percent of people survive, but these survivors typically have organ dysfunction, which may result in amputation. Treatment of DIC includes correcting the cause, intravenous fluids, transfusion of platelets, clotting factors (fresh frozen plasma), blood, and fibrinogen. My father was now in the ICU in critical condition and the doctors were very clear that the only hope was this "miracle," and his recovery was looking dismal. He had so many hurdles to climb to just become "stable."

The news was grave, and over the next forty-eight hours my father received 150 pints of blood products into his body. Given that the human body holds between eight and twelve pints of blood on average, his system was replaced several times over. The physicians and nurses were amazing during this time, keeping us readily informed and abreast of each issue. The "issues" become complicated when the delicate balance between normal and abnormal is disrupted, causing a cascade of events that now began to impact every system of the perfectly designed human body. While we prepared for the worst and the situation remained grim, we continued to pray and hope for the best outcome. Though he had a very low chance of survival, we clung to the hope that he would possibly pull through, knowing that the physicians and nursing staff were doing all they could and perhaps it was not "his time." We knew he was walking a very thin line between life and death. My mother would listen to the physician's daily update and seek clarification if needed, so we were constantly on top of each and every issue as it evolved or resolved.

I vividly remember people spilling out of the waiting room while there supporting our entire family. The community of support was amazing; there is power in support. Food, drinks, blankets, and any other commodity you could think of were brought in for us as we were not going anywhere while our father was in the midst of the fight of his life. We spent several nights in the waiting room, and any chance we got to see Dad, we would go sit with him, speak positive words of encouragement, and just hold his hands. In the ICU, visits are brief and carefully monitored by the staff for the benefit of the sick patient.

My mother has always been a strong woman of faith, and while she was praying for her husband to survive, she also understood that these could be his last hours. She was cautiously optimistic yet realistic and honest about every detail. She comforted us during this uncertain time but also told us that our father may not survive. While my father could not respond due to sedation and tubes coming out from all over his body, we were assured that he COULD hear us as hearing is one of the last senses to go. So, my mom told my father we were all OK and that she loved him and was grateful for him. This is a process of letting your loved one know that no matter what the outcome of the situation, you have given them permission to "go" and release them from the burden of worrying about you. This becomes the delicate dance between staying hopeful and remaining sensitive to my father's emotional state that he cannot address due to his critical condition.

On day five, my father's surgeon said that he would need to go into surgery again, but that this could not happen until he was more stable, and he was truly uncertain that this would actually occur. Dad was still bleeding internally. The doctor described the surgery as going in and tying off the bleeders that were continuing to ooze blood into my father's body, especially in his stomach where just days before the previous surgery was completed. This now became our focus: for Dad to have a slight improvement in his condition so he could withstand another surgery. The next morning the doctor came to us and said, "There's been a very, very small change in your father's blood counts, so we are going into surgery immediately." A cheer went up from our family and friends in the waiting room. Progress! The doctor, of course, told us that this was a high-risk procedure, and if Dad made it through, he could experience a myriad of complications. He also explained that due to the fragility of my father, they would need to operate on him in the Trendelenburg position, which is a position where a patient in shock (due to excessive blood loss) lies face-up on the operating table, which is purposely tilted such that the head is lower than the feet. This allows blood perfusion to the brain through the use of gravity and also assists in the filling and distention of the upper central veins. But given the situation, we were willing to allow the doctors to try it, so they whisked my father off to the operating room (another moment where I wondered if I would see my dad alive again). As the complications continued to compound, my family sank deeper and deeper into despair. Yet despair was not an emotion my mother would let cloud her mind; she clung to her positivity and faith and encouraged us to be optimistic, as Dad was in the operating room and that alone was miraculous progress. I know that even his physicians were amazed by his ongoing core strength and determination.

Several hours later, my father arrived on the gurney in the ICU trailed by his physicians, who seemed to be breathing a sigh of relief. He had made it through and was alive. I don't think anything could have prepared us for the sight we were then about to see. My father was almost unrecognizable. He was not a big man to begin with, but he came back from the operating room with his head completely engorged and so grotesquely large that his chin was resting on his nipples. Imagine a Fred Flintstone head. But, he was alive!! Even the doctors were astonished; perhaps there was a miracle in the making. It was apparent by the entourage in the waiting room just how large a support system my dad had, and at some level, he became encouraged by the combination of their energy and his drive to survive.

The surgery was successful, the bleeding had finally subsided, and his blood counts began to normalize. Over time his head came back to its normal size, and the doctors were amazed as they watched my father slowly improve. They had truly been instrumental in facilitating this miracle, and the renewed hope that my dad might now recover began to bubble up within us all.

At one point, when I was at the bedside with my father, who was now alert, I turned to him and asked him how he was coping with all that he had been through. To me it seemed that he was suffering and was having to endure so many traumas to his body. He scrunched up his face and only said, "It's rough." I grasped his hand as tears came down both our cheeks. I told him to keep fighting if he could, and that we were with him every step of the way.

Slowly, over the next several days, little bits of progress were detected and blood counts began to rise. The tubes began to disappear and the monitors stopped their continuous beeping. After two weeks, he was eventually moved off the ICU with only one tube attached to him. The only complication he developed was an abscess, a small swollen area that contains infection and pus, in his liver. This infection needed to be resolved, or it could potentially lead to a larger scale, potentially deadly infection known as sepsis. This required a small procedure in the radiology department to insert a tube from his liver to the outside of his skin to allow for drainage of the abscess and to flush it from the outside.

This is where my hands-on advocacy role started, and my mother was at the helm as she taught me that proper sterile technique would be the next hurdle to make certain that this was done properly. If not, the chances of infection were high and we could not chance infection and potential sepsis after all that my father had been through. We were educated on how to do this, and we quickly realized that a drainage tube from the liver was not something that the hospital staff was adept at handling themselves, so we made arrangements with the staff for us to be responsible to perform this procedure each day ourselves with their oversight. With staff turnover between shifts, and the inability to always communicate effectively between the shifts, my mother and I made ourselves available each day that this needed to be done, and six weeks later, my father was released home with no abscess and no apparent residual complications from this harrowing experience. By all accounts a true miracle! He recovered both physically and mentally from this arduous medical event.

Once home, I asked my father, just like I did in the early days of the ICU, "How are you coping with everything you have been through?" His response was shocking, but one I would hear over and over from other patients: "I really don't remember much of it." He seemed to have a built-in amnesia to protect him from the trauma of all he had experienced.

Upon discharge, his strength was understandably diminished. He and my mother started a daily exercise program as part of his physical therapy until they could walk the neighborhood. He recovered so well over the next four weeks that he returned to his job at IBM. His abscess was healed, his diabetes was stable, and though weak, he was very close to his baseline status.

Though he had built-in amnesia, I did not. And although it is now thirty-two years later, I have vivid memories of my father and some of what he said to me and how he looked. These don't haunt me, but rather I reflect with gratitude not only for his life but for what he taught me through this experience. I was dating Steve at the time (who is now my husband) and going through this crisis together definitely expedited our dating journey, as the emotions during a time like that were real and raw. Nine months later, my father walked me down the aisle at our wedding, and as I grasped his arm, I was filled with emotion about what this moment meant; it was overwhelming and I still feel the same emotion of grasping his arm on that day. I knew to never take a day for granted, and the fact that he was there for my wedding day is a gift for which I will forever be grateful.

Outcome:

After six weeks in the hospital and four weeks at home to recover, my father returned to work at IBM in Bethesda, Maryland, and retired three years later in good health and on his own terms. He continued with routine medical care and continued to manage his diabetes with diet, exercise, and stable blood sugars.

He walked this grateful daughter down the aisle nine months after this health crisis. He lived fifteen quality years beyond this near-fatal medical crisis, attended all five of his children's weddings, and was there to celebrate the birth of ten out of fifteen grandchildren. Up until his last breath, he had a good quality of life. He relished his life extension as did his favorite nurse, my mother, and his second favorite nurse, me. As a father, he taught me well and enriched my life in every way.

The start of my advocacy journey:

I learned a great deal from this initial experience that stuck with me. My mother became my mentor and had me come along beside her and learn how to navigate difficult health journeys.

Through this experience, my mom taught me:

- not to give up hope despite desperate circumstances
- prayers can be answered
- focus on the big things in life, not the small stuff
- lean on family, friends, and community in times of need and then return the favor when others are in need
- (Having our "village's" support was vital in meeting our physical needs while our mental attention was focused on our sick family member. Their ability to feed us, provide a shoulder to cry on, and run endless errands while we were in the hospital was pivotal for us to continue focusing on Dad and remaining alert to the crisis du jour.)

- how to react to a health crisis in a pragmatic fashion and not overreact emotionally
- always err on the side of positivity and optimism
- focus on gratitude each step of the way; it minimizes the insults
- listen well; listen to what the medical team tells you, and verify that the information being passed between team members is accurate and precise
- in the event that there is misinformation, gently inquire and clarify in a non-threatening way
- get copies of labs, diagnostic tests, and other important documents to avoid any miscommunication at any given time when dealing with the medical experts
- trust health care professionals but ask open-ended questions and don't feel intimidated by doing so

As a result of my time spent invested in my father's difficult situation in 1988, I was now launched into a world of fascinating experiences that were not only tedious and arduous but also exhilarating at the same time.

Advocacy tips:

- Knowledge is power, and the more you know the more you can help others understand their particular situation. In cases where you don't have the knowledge, seek it, research it, and look for answers.
- Many times in my career I have been faced with situations that seemed extremely grim with no ability to see into the future. I learned with each experience to be hopeful and cautiously optimistic.
- Be educated but never give up hope.
- Empowering people to navigate difficult health journeys is frightening but satisfying.
- Help others find answers, investigate, and find the best path for you, your friend, or your loved one.
- Seek pathways that provide options while supporting the patient as they overcome obstacles; stay optimistic and supportive, and be their voice when they can no longer vocalize.

This is called health advocacy.

· Chapter 2 ·

Glioblastoma and a Groom

"Calmness of mind is one of the beautiful jewels of wisdom."

—James Allen

Dan, my husband's only sibling, was a thirty-year-old pediatric licensed clinical social worker (LCSW) living the good life in Atlanta. In September 1997, Steve and I were in Atlanta for his wedding to a beautiful woman from Georgia named Audrey. She was from a wonderful, loving family, and family was important to both the bride and groom. They first met in Ohio and then dated for several years while Audrey was in law school. As we were scurrying about getting ready for the big event, he mentioned to my husband and me that he was having pain around his neck, telling us he thought he had pulled a muscle. He had numbness and tingling down his right arm. His remedy was to get massages, which he was doing routinely in the days prior to the wedding. At the time, we did not think too much about this possible pinched nerve, and we carried on with the joyous celebration.

The wedding was a blast. The ceremony and reception were as beautiful and special as they could be. We danced, we toasted, and we celebrated for days. They had met their soul mates, and we were thrilled with our new sister-in-law.

Three weeks later, in early October, we were on a family bicycling trip through the beautiful Shenandoah Valley when we got a call from Dan. He proceeded to tell us that he had double vision, and it seemed to be getting worse very quickly. My heart skipped a beat, as I had just been through a similar situation with my best friend and her brother. These symptoms drew red flags in my mind: pain down the arm, numbness, tingling, and now double vision. Could this be a brain tumor? Of course, I told him to call and get seen ASAP by a neurologist, but he told me that he had tried, but his managed care health insurance had an eight-week waiting list. With these worrisome symptoms, I felt waiting eight weeks was not an option, and my advocacy brain kicked into gear. I told him to go to the emergency room after 5 p.m. They went to the ER around 9 p.m. after their Friday night family dinner and got the results of the scan at 4 a.m.: Dan had a brain tumor. They called and told us the news and his difficult journey began. He had only been married three weeks and still had yet to celebrate his honeymoon. At the sound of this news, I felt desperation and pessimism about the possible outcome, but I knew from past experience that I had to focus on hope. I realized that Dan was one of the most optimistic people I knew, so I took his lead.

In Dan's case, his wife was his primary advocate and did an incredible job. We were family support, and since she was a lawyer and knew how to effectively research any topic, she would bounce things off of me, and we would devise plans of how we were going to help Dan fight this. From the beginning, he said that he did not want any statistics or details of the fatality of this disease discussed with him as he was only concerned about staying positive and leaving the gory details to his wife. This agreement worked for them, and they had a plan. Audrey was as proactive as she could be. She researched every article she could find in order to educate herself as much as possible for her groom. It was the perfect combination as he was so optimistic and she was so thorough in her research.

Within ten days, a biopsy was scheduled through his managed care insurance plan, and we all flew to Atlanta to support the two of them. The doctor emerged from the operating room very optimistic. He felt very sure that this lesion was a "cyst" and was not cancerous "by the looks of it" in the operating room. He sent the pathology out to various notable institutions, and the results came back about ten days later with a malignant finding from each of the different sites. Despite this information, the doctor still felt compelled to believe it was not accurate. He then requested a review of the slides from two more institutions.

The delay in a firm diagnosis resulted in Dan not seeing an oncologist for over four weeks. As it turned out, the tumor was, in fact, malignant and was described as an oligodendroglioma. The Cleveland Clinic defines this extremely rare type of mass as "an uncommon tumor that forms in either the frontal or temporal lobes of the brain, but in rare cases can form in the spinal cord. It develops from cells called oligodendrocytes which create a substance that protects nerves in the brain and helps them to function." During the four-week delay, the tumor had started to grow "tentacles" and treatment needed to be started as soon as possible.

However, since the oncologist that Dan was assigned to in his managed care insurance plan was a general oncologist, not an oncologist that specialized in brain tumors, Audrey wanted him to see an oncologist who solely focused on brain tumors, specifically oligodendrogliomas and glioblastomas. Her search started, but they faced many hurdles as Dan's insurance plan did not have a specialist like this in his plan, and his coverage was rejected for going "out of network." Audrey swung into action and asked for all of our help. She figured the more involvement, the more momentum.

Audrey took the lead on this in Atlanta, and we helped fight the cause from Maryland and made this effort into a national campaign to get Dan the treatment he needed and deserved. Her efforts led to a petition, and we involved as many people as we could to get what we felt was "the standard of care" for Dan. While we appreciated the intent of managed care insurance plans, we felt that when faced with a health care issue they could not adequately treat, they should provide coverage for an "out of network" option. Among all of us, thousands of people signed the petition, including those in positions of power. We finally got approved for Dan to see a top expert in the field of oncology and brain tumors. This was an extremely arduous task, but because Audrey made it happen, her groom now had a medical expert in place to help him face his own personal Mt. Everest. Audrey stepped up and executed the plan in the best way possible.

Though his care was delayed, the fight was victorious, and Dan got excellent care from top experts, including physicians, nurses, infusion center professionals, and hospitals. Audrey made sure that her husband was able to get the best treatment available which included chemotherapy and radiation.

He and Audrey worked as a great team. They fought this fight together with spunk and laughter. Their newlywed life started off with this major roadblock, but they both chose to focus on the silver lining and they lived life as well as they could, meeting up with friends, going out to dinner, attending Friday night family dinners, watching movies at home, and whatever else Dan felt up to doing. Audrey made it happen. They were an amazing duo and his optimism helped fuel her passion to keep pressing on in a positive way.

His care and treatment were top-notch, and he was able to live a relatively normal life for three and a half years thanks to his wife's research and diligence. During his illness, Dan wrote an article about fighting cancer, and even wrote a book about diversity and inclusion called *The Cats of Inman Park*. He surpassed the average survival rate of seventeen months, and while he did experience some side effects from his chemotherapy, he chose to live a life of hope and to keep focusing on living. He did eventually go on a wonderful honeymoon with his wife. He traveled to Israel and to the Grand Canyon. The cover of this book was a photo that Dan took while hiking in the Canyon (2000) and has always been one of my favorites. He was determined to optimize his time and focus on what he had to live for and do things that he had always wanted to do. He did not focus on life expectancy or "what happens if." He truly never looked at the data that predicted life expectancies; he left that to us, his support team. We were constantly updated by Audrey and Dan, made some brief trips to see them, and Dan even carved out time to spend with each of his two older nephews so they could get to know each other. These trips are still a great memory for both my sons, Matthew and Christopher. He was selfless and had an invigorating personality. We continued to cling to hope and marveled at how far Dan had come, defying all the odds of his disease.

In June of 2001, it became apparent that he was starting to struggle. His gait was unsteady, his vision was affected and it was getting harder for him to live his typical life, but he never wavered from focusing on the positives. As part of his advocacy team, we met with Audrey and came up with a plan that would offer more family support for Dan and Audrey. Since we lived several states away, we had to devise a plan to make this work for them and also be there when they needed us. We took off work and made a schedule to go help one week at a time. As a family, we opted to split up the weeks and take turns going to Atlanta to help them. The family team consisted of me, Steve, and Leah, Steve and Dan's mother. I went first and spent an amazing week with them, taking him to appointments and taking him out and about, especially to nice restaurants since this was most important to him. Because of his physical limitations, he took pleasure in a few precious things, and food became a primary focus. Each morning, he loved deciding where we would go eat that day. His gait was becoming increasingly unsteady, and there were times that I was concerned that he would fall when we were together, but I am so glad we ventured out. Once he almost toppled off the porch, and my heart dropped to my stomach thinking how close a call that was. But regardless of any of the negatives, it was such a blessing to spend time with Dan and Audrey, and I marveled at their strength and positive attitude. Dan continued to live his life with humor, and laughter was an important part of his day.

After my week, Steve came down to stay with his brother and sister-in-law. One evening, we had the opportunity to sit down and discuss next steps. We decided that when Dan was unable to be cared for at home, he would go to an inpatient hospice facility nearby in Atlanta.

When a patient is at the end of their life, they have multiple options: They can stay home, typically with twenty-four-hour hired care if the home is set up for it and the family opts for this, or they can go to a facility where hospice services can be brought to the facility. They can also go to a hospice-owned facility, which is what Dan and Audrey decided to do. It was so helpful to have discussed this ahead of time and to then have a plan to follow. Good friends of Dan and Audrey's took it upon themselves to visit various facilities and report back about what they thought was the best place for Dan. We were fortunate to have that level of support.

We continued to rotate weeks, and eventually, the whole family came to Atlanta for Dan's last days.

The one "gift" cancer seems to give is time. This time can be well spent and productive, as it was in this case. We got to complete any unfinished business as much as it was possible to do, we had beautiful meaningful conversations, we laughed, we talked, and we ate and ate and ate. The hospice facility commented that they never had a hospice patient eat as much as Dan. He would wake up in the morning, decide what he wanted to eat that day, and his care team would scramble to make it happen. Because he had many friends, he had hundreds of visitors who came to the facility to say goodbye. He would tell jokes and ask me to tell funny stories about his nephews (my sons), and we would laugh until we cried. I witnessed a beautiful wife prepare for a life without her thirty-four-year-old husband as she paved the most beautiful road that she could for him. She was selfless, focused, and determined to do everything and anything she could for her husband, and she did it well.

Outcome:

Dan lived three and a half years with his brain tumor and led a busy life despite his illness. In his last ten days, Dan was in a hospice facility, and it became a rotating door day and night for friends from far and wide. It was almost a party-like atmosphere for him as he was shown love by so many. Then, forty-eight hours before his death, when he slipped into unconsciousness, his appetite finally left him, and he closed his eyes. Dan's life was brief, but very well lived. Steve and Dan had several meaningful discussions about the end of life, leaving no stone unturned. Dan verbalized satisfaction with his life filled with humor, deep friendships, an amazing wife, and no regrets. His brief life was chock full of accomplishments, and in his thirty-four years he did as much as an eighty-four-year-old; his life was compacted yet beautiful and he effected change in others through his career counseling children; he was a loving brother, son, uncle, and a loving, doting husband.

Advocacy tips from "Top 10 Things to Remember When Fighting Brain Cancer!" By Dan Kohn:

Before he died, Dan wrote a blog post containing ten advocacy tips for helping someone with cancer. You can read the full blog here.

Find an advocate who can gather information: Audrey did this for Dan.

Allow supportive friends and family to help, and surround yourself with them: We took turns staying with Dan.

Fight for a doctor that you believe in, a doctor who believes that they can help you: Audrey refused to take no for an answer and moved mountains to get the right doctor for Dan.

Keep a sense of humor: Dan showed us how to do this very well.

Find a support group: Dan and Audrey did this with their friends and through a cancer-survivor support group where they met amazing people. We found support in our life group who "carried" us through this very difficult chapter of our family's life.

Find joy in your day: Dan and Audrey modeled this. Dan used to walk through the neighborhood taking pictures and videotaping interviews with random people. When his wife would come home from work, Dan would showcase his adventures for her.

Keep in mind that you are not a victim; you are a survivor.

Do not get clinically depressed: take an anti-depressant, because clinical depression has physical manifestations that contribute to your already difficult situation. Use tools to help, and know that there is no shame in getting some pharmaceutical assistance.

Strengthen your spirit: Dan sought out his relationship with God, explored his faith, began praying regularly, and realized he wasn't as afraid of death as he once thought. He never took his Judaism seriously before this time of his life.

Be kind to yourself for giving into cravings: Decadron=grease+sugar+fried+chocolate+four inches on your waistline. Dan's cravings were intense. Though his wife was not thrilled with his choices sometimes—she tried to get him to eat a healthy diet—he regularly ate donuts and fried chicken. Sometimes his friends snuck him contraband. Dan sometimes felt that he had so little pleasure that these foods gave him temporary relief. Audrey continued her efforts, and ultimately turned a blind eye toward his indulgences. It was impossible to deprive Dan of anything that brought him joy, even if it was being found in king-sized candy bars.

· Chapter 3 ·

Come Pick Me Up

"Sometimes all you have to do is be quiet and listen, stay present and calm amid the storms, be the energy of love rather than trying to corral it."

—Brendon Burchard

I got a call on a beautiful summer evening from Leah, my mother-in-law. She was a well-respected teacher with lots of energy and sass. She taught at our local high school in the English department and was the yearbook advisor for many award-winning yearbooks. Since she taught at the same school her sons attended, they had some fun stories. The sons remember dodging her in the hallways so they wouldn't be seen. But most people didn't want to dodge her because she has always been the life of the party and a party all by herself.

She told me that she was walking up the sidewalk to see her neighbor when she tripped and fell, landing on the cement. After being taken to the hospital, she learned she had shattered her pelvis and dislodged her hip prosthesis in the process. She was being evaluated in the ER and would call us when she got to her room as it was obvious that she was going to be admitted to the orthopedic wing for evaluation and possible surgery.

She was admitted to the hospital, and the orthopedic surgeon was coming to evaluate her in the morning to put an action plan of care together for Leah. She was in excruciating pain due to the pelvic fracture.

> Because the pelvic bone is large and contains a rich blood supply, these fractures are extremely painful due to the bleeding into the surrounding tissues. Heavy doses of pain medication are required to control the pain for these patients. They are unable to bear weight, they must stay in bed, and all activities of daily living are done in the bed, prompting more pain with movement and turning.

The next morning I got a call from Leah telling me that she was discharged and wanted to know if I could pick her up. Discharged? I was shocked because the information provided the night before was such that a discharge so soon the very next day did not make sense. She proceeded to tell me that the orthopedic surgeon had evaluated her case and concluded that the damage was too vast to perform the surgery at our local community hospital, so she would need to go to a trauma center to have surgery in the "near future," but in the interim, she would be discharged home. The discharge orders were written, and she was letting me know.

I was unclear how this would happen. Leah was bedbound, not ambulatory, had a shattered pelvis, and was in tremendous pain. She could not possibly ride in a car. How would I go and "pick her up"? She said she didn't know, but this is what the nurse told her and she needed to go.

I hung up the phone and told her that I would call her back once I figured out how to facilitate the request from the doctor and, ultimately, the nurse. I could not figure out how this situation could lead to a discharge on that day. So I called the nurse and told her that their request seemed unreasonable, not to mention unsafe and nearly impossible, so the physician and hospital staff needed to rethink the discharge for Leah. I asked some important questions about mobility, Leah's safety, and how we would struggle to safely meet the request. The nurse agreed that this seemed like a complicated situation and followed up with the physician who had written the order to discuss our concerns.

Luckily, they rescinded the discharge, and she was kept in the local community hospital for several days. Then, when it was safe to do so, given the instability of the fracture, she was transferred to a high-level trauma center in Washington, DC.

However, at the higher-level hospital, she ran into some potential issues on her own, and thankfully, she was of sound mind to recognize them. The first issue she ran into was that she noticed that her ID wrist band was for the wrong patient. She was mixed up with another patient, so she was being treated for that person's health issues and not the fractured pelvis that she actually had. Secondly, the X-rays at the bedside were for another patient, and thirdly, she was placed on a commode for an extended period of time without access to the call light and needed to yell loudly to eventually be helped. These mix-ups did not bring Leah or her family much comfort and we soon realized that one of us should be with her to avoid any further issues.

She was eventually operated on and, at the appropriate point in her recovery, was sent to a rehabilitation center and then home.

The request for discharge was illogical. Thankfully, as a nurse, I was able to reconcile this before I went to the hospital and put Leah and me in a dangerous situation. I feel for those who are not medical and do not know they have a voice to speak up when something doesn't seem right. We need to all know that knowledge is power and feel empowered to ask questions. Fortunately, Medicare and most insurance companies allow for an appeal process if you feel your loved one is being discharged prematurely, and we have advised clients to use this tactic on many occasions when a discharge felt inappropriate.

Outcome:

The patient successfully got transferred to a higher-level medical institution to get medical care that could not be provided at the local community hospital. Luckily, the nurse understood she was being put into a potentially harmful situation by having an unsafe premature discharge. She got top-notch medical care and recovered nicely from the surgery and returned to her baseline prior to any further injury occurring.

She is currently eighty-two years old and living a healthy, vibrant life enjoying family and retirement to the max at the beach in a large retirement community. She has taken her own advocacy very seriously and has learned from this experience.

Advocacy tips:

- It is OK to ask questions and intervene on the patient's behalf if you have permission to do so.
- Do not feel intimidated by asking these questions or asking for clarification; it can have a positive impact.
- If the staff doesn't verify your medical bracelet before working on you, make sure you check it yourself. The danger here is in a situation where the patient has dementia or some other medical condition that diminishes their awareness, insight, or judgement, which is why we often recommend another person stay with these types of clients to add a level of security and safety.

· Chapter 4 ·

The Lyme Mystery

*"Flow with whatever may happen and let your mind be free:
Stay centered by accepting whatever you are doing. This is the
ultimate."*

—Chuang Tzu

In January of 2007, our seven-year-old son, Michael,
began exhibiting strange behaviors. Initially, each action
was explained away by either my husband or me with
some seemingly rational explanation. He began having
temper tantrums, insomnia, headaches, lethargy, night

terrors, mood swings, weight gain, and multiple complaints of aches and pains. We continued to not make a big deal about each of these symptoms and continued to rationalize them away: "Oh, he was up late on Saturday," "He went to bed too late," or "He went to a birthday party and maybe ate too much sugar," and on and on the excuses flowed. Yet, his problems continued. He would stand beside our bed in the middle of the night telling us he could not sleep. He would get up and run through the house screaming in terror that he was being chased or some other irrational delusion. But during the day, he became a couch potato. He would cry and mope and lie around day and night, extremely moody and unhappy for no particular reason. On top of that, he had stomach aches, headaches, joint pains, back pains, and finger pain. He started missing school because he did not feel well on most days. If he did get to school, they would call me to come get him because of one complaint or another. He began to gain weight and suddenly he was up forty-five pounds in one year. My older sons were tired of us making excuses for why Michael didn't feel well and, at one point, felt that he was just badly behaved and should be disciplined accordingly. Additionally, I was in graduate school so I was under quite a bit of stress personally.

Prior to this, he was a happy, well-adjusted youngest child of three boys. He would always go with the flow of whatever was going on in the house. He would go with us to all of his brothers' sporting events, and he was always good natured and made friends easily with other youngsters he met at ballgames or at the park.

His situation just didn't make any sense. That's when suddenly one day I realized that something was going on with my son: Michael was sick.

In August of 2007, we were on a family vacation at the beach with another family. By now, we were somewhat used to his complaining and took it all in stride. As we were preparing to go out to dinner to grab some burgers at the local burger joint, he was lying on the couch and said, "Bring something home for me please." I looked at my husband and said something is definitely wrong. What eight-year-old does not want to grab a burger at the beach unless something is really wrong with him? This was my "aha" moment, and I knew I needed to investigate further. I was not going to relent in my quest for the truth . . . something was wrong. After eight months of this, I was starting to connect the dots with these symptoms. I needed to find out what had changed my healthy, happy, active child into a miserable, complaining, moody boy. I needed to find out exactly what it was and help my son.

Realizing there was a problem, I could not wait to get home to see our pediatrician. When we got home, I made an appointment. Now empowered by my studies toward an advanced degree, I told the doctor about my son's myriad of symptoms and asked him what he thought could be the cause. I was hoping that he could tie all of this together for us and come up with a diagnosis. I think the doctor thought

I was just a stressed-out mom who was making a big deal out of nothing. I tried to sum up how different our son had become over the previous eight months and expressed my concern for this change. It was hard for us as a family, but for Michael, it was worse: he was living a miserable life over which he seemed to have no control. I asked the doctor for a workup to include a liver enzyme panel, kidney function tests, thyroid panel, a workup for diabetes and a Lyme titer just to cover all bases. I was told they would run the test, but the pediatrician specifically said, "This is definitely not Lyme."

A week later the doctor called me back to tell me all the tests were normal and the Lyme titer was not back, but he was certain that was not the problem. This left me puzzled as to what should be my next step, until twenty-four hours later when he called me back and told me that the Lyme titer was positive and "very positive at that!" The doctor was shocked as he told me the presentation of symptoms was unlike any Lyme presentation he had seen. I was thrilled just to have an answer and a potential solution, since Lyme is treatable. Because Doxycycline was not recommended for children under ten years of age, Michael was placed on Amoxicillin. Over the course of the next three weeks, our son returned to his baseline behavior that we had not seen in over eight months. He was happy, not complaining; he slept well; he became active again; he ate regular meals; he did not wake up and stand at my bedside every night whining that he couldn't sleep, and we were so grateful to have him back. After twenty-one days, the antibiotic course was completed, and we went on about our lives as if the problem was solved.

Within three weeks after completing the antibiotics, Michael again began to feel poorly and many of his symptoms began to return. Six weeks after completing the antibiotic therapy, Michael was back to feeling terrible and we went back to the pediatrician's office. I needed guidance and direction for how to get my son help. We met with the doctor, and he was stumped, as he looked up CDC guidelines and they only recommended a three-week course of antibiotics for Lyme disease. He called a pediatric infectious disease specialist at Children's Hospital in Washington, DC, and was told there is nothing more that could be done for him. They said, "Lyme is acute and antibiotics are only recommended for twenty-one days. There must be another explanation for what is going on with the child. He may need a psychiatrist." Our pediatrician was sorry he could not offer us any more help; I left the office very disheartened but knew I needed to figure out how to help my son. I was on a mission to get answers for Michael and get him back to his healthy baseline.

As a mother and a nurse, it was unacceptable to allow my child to suffer like this. How could I accept that my perfectly normal eight-year-old felt this ill and I should just accept it as, "Oh well, that is just the way it is." But that is what I was advised by our pediatrician, who had been treating all three of my children since birth. Thus began the search for a doctor to help us. I did research, I called colleagues, I read articles and finally found a local physician who treated Lyme and said he could help my son. Again, Michael was started on a course of multiple antibiotics, probiotics, and some vitamin supplements. Again, he started to feel better, but when his liver enzymes began to elevate, I was concerned. I was working in a GI practice at the time and knew that elevated liver enzymes meant liver inflammation, and this was not good. I conferred with the doctor, and we cut back on some of his medications and his liver enzymes returned to normal. But we were on a roller coaster ride, and I soon found out how controversial, unpredictable, and elusive Lyme disease could be. The physician treating Michael told me he was under a microscope at all times, being repeatedly investigated by the State Department of Health. As a mother, I was so grateful that a physician would treat this illness that our own pediatrician could not help us with. We now had been watching our son suffer on a daily basis and basically missed out on two years of his life while he lay on the couch watching the world go on around him.

In 2009, I was referred to a local anesthesiologist who had a homeopathic medicine practice right down the street. I credit this physician with restoring Michael's life to a more normal place. He allowed Michael to go on with his life and enabled him to quit all prescription medications and get on with living symptom free. While the world of homeopathy was new to me, I soon became a big fan. I have since referred hundreds of people to this physician from all over the world and have seen amazing results. Michael slowly got back to baseline as all his aches and pains began to subside. He was able to sleep, get involved again with sports, and play outside. His mood was happy, no crying spells, and he was able to regularly attend school. Thankfully, he was able to have healthy active years during high school. He competed in athletics and was social and outgoing.

Not a day goes by that I am not grateful that my son is now twenty-one years old, happy, healthy, pain free, and is even a Division 1 collegiate student athlete. He has come all this way thanks to pushing and researching for a solution and by not taking no for an answer. I insisted on pressing the medical system to get him the treatment he needed. One of the many benefits of residing in a major metropolitan area is the access to medical options "off the grid" that can be so helpful when mainstream medicine does not have answers. Homeopathy has been the adjunctive therapy that helped our son improve his life and provided solutions that have optimized his life.

I do believe that the "benefit" of Michael being sick as a child allowed me to recognize these unusual symptoms of Lyme in hundreds of people who had suffered for years without explanation. Since becoming a NP in 2007, I have been able to diagnose these unusual symptoms in people. I don't believe these things happen without good reason. This ability to "think outside the box" has helped improve people's lives when there seemed to be no other answer. I am also eternally grateful to Dr. S, who not only changed Michael's life but has impacted thousands of patients for the good.

Outcome:

After high school, Michael took a post-graduate year to become more prepared physically, mentally, and emotionally for college. He studied at a boarding school in Florida that offered college classes and a very rigorous baseball routine before applying to college the spring after his senior year.

He stands just under 6'5" and is 225 pounds. He has been able to stay healthy and strong and still sees the holistic physician who treated him for Lyme. On occasion, he can still present with unexplained anxiety or difficulty sleeping that is related to his history of Lyme. He still gets treatment on an ongoing basis. I am so proud of Michael for pressing on during some very hard years that he did not allow to shape his life. He has continued to work hard and be devoted, despite the many challenges he has faced, and truly rarely complained. From being sick for five years to achieving what he has been able to do takes fortitude and courage, I admire him for this accomplishment.

Advocacy tips:

Advocating for Michael was difficult because the pediatrician could not embrace what was wrong with our son and did not offer any solutions. To this day, people will question if in fact he truly had Lyme. I still have his lab tests from two years in a row which clearly show that this was the case.

- Do not rationalize away symptoms like we did.
- If you feel there is a medical reason for a certain behavior, don't give up until you find an answer.
- Tapping into resources can help you get answers. When you do this, you find out that you are not alone in your quest for certain information and there is strength in numbers. On our street of six homes, five of them have had a family member with Lyme disease. We have been able to network and support each other through our struggles while our loved ones got better. This was not a short journey for any of us.

embrace the "no regrets" philosophy for everyone, and this picture is different for each person facing end of life.

> "Do everything" means that in the event of a cardiac or respiratory arrest, they want their parents to have whatever measures are needed to keep them alive. This includes cardiopulmonary resuscitation (CPR), artificial ventilation, tube feeding, dialysis, IVs and any medications or fluids needed to sustain their lives.
>
> Each person gets to paint their own "canvas" or write their own final chapter the best they can. This is another reason why end-of-life conversations are imperative. Knowing where a loved one stands regarding their advanced directives helps guide care providers in cases of emergency and illness.
>
> Oftentimes, an attorney working on a Last Will and Testament can get a person to pen their own advanced directives at the same time. These directives often include specific instructions on medical care with a Living Will designed to ensure that when this person is unable to communicate, their wishes are carried out by medical providers.

We met this family in the fall of 2006, a mother and father married for sixty-five years, beginning to decline and needing help for eight hours a day. Mom was slipping a bit more than Dad. She was getting a bit unsteady, and they were having a hard time keeping up with the day-to-day chores of their large farmhouse in Virginia. The grandchildren checked in on them regularly and helped with errands and chores until the point when they felt they needed to bring in some additional help. The mom was not as able-bodied as she once was, and the dad was overwhelmed caring for the property, himself, and now his wife. The children sat them down and they hesitantly agreed to have us come on and help them part-time in their home.

My initial assessment was done, and I noted that they needed some grab bars for safety in the bathroom, in the shower, and next to the toilet. I requested all throw rugs, which are the main cause of falls in the elderly, be removed. I also suggested removing some clutter and furniture for better access and mobility for Mr. and Mrs. C. A customized care plan was written for the Cs, reviewed with the assigned caregivers, and then executed for our clients as we began services.

The caregivers helped with chores, meals, showers, light housekeeping, and medication reminders, and soon a nice rapport was established with Mr. and Mrs. C. By March, Mrs. C became weak and needed to be hospitalized and then moved on to a rehabilitation center. Our caregivers were splitting their time between the rehabilitation center and the family home where Mr. C was living. He was still able to do some activities of daily living on his own but required more assistance with meals and chores around the home than when we initially started services.

Once we are on a job and providing caregiver services, we have found that taking the caregiver with the patient to the different levels of care hastens the healing process for the patient and helps them meet their goals faster after an acute medical setback. The caregiver is like their own personal cheerleader who already has experience with the specific nuances of their patient and the added benefit of safety in the hospital where patients tend to get confused and have an increased chance of falling in unfamiliar surroundings. Short-staffed hospitals and rehabilitation centers always welcome the extra set of hands that a private caregiver can add, as their ratio can be upwards of 1:10 staff to patients. The extra eyes and ears also provide peace of mind to families after they leave their loved one, as they are not alone. I have done the same with my own family members since 1988 when my father was sick. When families cannot be with their loved one in the hospital, they often opt to hire a caregiver to be at the bedside to minimize the opportunity for preventable incidents.

A patient used to a private caregiver can experience difficulty when taken to medical facilities without their caregiver. In an unfamiliar setting, like a rehab center, they see a lot of new faces, which definitely complicates the situation for clients who are used to the same three to four faces in a week.

While Mr. C was OK with the additional services, Mrs. C had a harder time adjusting in the rehabilitation center. For someone like Mrs. C, who was used to having someone help her promptly when she needed to go to the bathroom, having to wait for her call bell to be answered caused a delay to the point where she became impatient trying to refrain from voiding, which led her to become incontinent. The delays in receiving timely assistance also increased her anxiety. At one point she became impulsive and got up by herself only to fall to the floor, further complicating her recovery. This is frustrating for patients who aren't used to waiting to get help. Experience has taught us that many folks who go into a hospital or rehabilitation facility continent actually are discharged "incontinent," and on many occasions, I have heard medical personal say, "Just pee on the pad. We will clean it up." This is easier said than done for patients who are simply not comfortable with voiding or defecating on themselves and then sitting in it until someone has the time to come and clean them up. It actually makes a patient feel worse on many levels and can often lengthen their recovery time, not to mention increase the opportunity for a urinary tract infection.

A decrease in appetite, weakness, and lethargy are all very typical for patients who have gone from home to the hospital and then to rehabilitation after an acute illness. It is very disruptive to our elderly clients' lives and often the food is not palatable, as they are used to home-cooked foods that they enjoy. Many patients recovering from illness tend to drop their nutritional status quickly, which results in low albumin levels. I like to pay close attention to this indicator as it provides information about how well a patient will heal and recover.

Monitoring albumin levels has been an efficient way for us to help our clients get better. In a facility, getting a dietician involved promptly can help remedy the situation. Typically nutritional supplements or protein powders administered daily help rectify the deficiency. If the albumin level drops precipitously and is not addressed, it can lead to a myriad of health concerns. One symptom includes the collection of fluid in the extremities, a condition known as "third spacing." Once this occurs, diuretics are typically used and the cascade of events stemming from this tends to multiply. The diuretics can cause dehydration, electrolyte imbalances, and ultimately kidney and other organ damage. One supplement that can help with low albumin is easy-to-find protein drinks such as "Ensure" or "Boost," and these products are readily available in multiple flavors and consistencies. You can choose between a dense milk-based shake product or a protein-packed clear juice product based on your preference.

We began increasing our staffing hours with the Cs as their need for help increased. Caregivers would train and orient the new caregivers, which helped the new staff more easily assimilate to the family's routine. This allowed them to learn the various nuances of care necessary to keep Mr. and Mrs. C comfortable and content.

In September 2007, Mr. C gradually became weaker and started to fall frequently. He went to the hospital where he was found to have a low sodium level and ended up staying for a week. His caregivers were at the hospital with him because he was fearful at night and was afraid to sleep, so by bringing in a caregiver, he was comfortable, which helped him to relax and sleep better. After his sodium levels normalized, he opted not to go to a rehabilitation center because he was more comfortable with the idea of going home. With home physical therapy, occupational therapy, and a nurse coming, he could get almost the same amount of care in familiar surroundings, and most importantly, Mrs. C was there to cheer him on. His care plan needed to be updated as he now required fluid restrictions, monitoring of his sodium level via routine lab draws, and changes in his medication doses. Low sodium levels can at first be very subtle in one's symptom presentation, but sudden episodes of withdrawal, weakness, and falls; acute onset depression; or odd behaviors can result. If the sodium level gets too low, seizures can result, and the situation can become grave quickly. Likewise, remedying the situation must be done slowly and carefully in the hospital to minimize other issues.

By November Mrs. C was in need of a rollator, which is a walker with wheels. She was unsteady and weak, and this device afforded her more stability. So a PT evaluated her and trained her in her home on its safe use. Not every patient is appropriate for a rollator. In some cases, a standard walker is better, which is why the decision about which device to use should be made by a trained PT.

Next, in March 2008, Mr. C had a cardiac event which required a visit to the ICU and the use of a respirator. His speech was affected, and he had many complications. The hospitalists and specialists in the hospital began to ask about advanced directives to help guide therapy for Mr. C, who was ninety years old at this time. The family had no doubt about what to do: "Do everything!" they said as they produced documentation to support full code status for their father. The hospital stay caused an increase in the acuity of Mr. C's care. At this time, he was now unable to walk, was on oxygen around the clock, and needed to be turned and repositioned every two hours to prevent bed sores.

> Because high-acuity patients don't always like to be turned, pressure sores occur more frequently in this group and can begin to happen within a twenty-four-hour period. Preventing pressure sores in a bedbound patient is a challenge but can be avoided with meticulous care. It is the nutritional status coupled with appropriate fluids and minimizing pressure to the bony prominences (places where bones protrude out and can get irritated) that allow for improved outcome. Patients don't always feel them when they first start. The wounds develop from the inside out, so when it actually

opens on the surface of the skin, the damage has already occurred on the inside. And all you see initially on the outside is a small, reddened area, so it is often easily overlooked without a thorough inspection. I put this potential issue in a patient's care plan so all staff members are aware of it as a possibility. Pressure sores require great effort and meticulous care along with adequate nutrition to fully heal. The most common areas where pressure wounds occur are the heels, hips, and sacral areas. Daily bathing and skin checks need to be part of routine exams for each at-risk patient whether at home, hospital, or in a rehabilitation center.

Fortunately, neither Mr. C nor Mrs. C ever developed pressure wounds through the seven years we provided services for them. They also were fortunate enough to maintain the same caregivers who worked with the couple for over seven years.

After a prolonged hospitalization and rehabilitation stay, Mr. C went home to be with his wife and caregivers. The care team now was enhanced to include a registered nurse (RN) from the Medicare home health team, oxygen support for Mr. C, certified nursing assistants (CNAs), licensed practical nurses (LPNs), other RNs, and a certified registered nurse practitioner (CRNP) from our company. The care plan was continually updated and the caregivers were educated on how to care for Mr. C in his debilitated condition. A hospital bed was brought into the bedroom but Mr. and Mrs. C were still together in the same room, just as they wanted to be. Some urinary tract infections, falls, and a few minor infections were added to Mr. C's list of diagnoses, but he always managed to pull through his ailments. There were times when the C home felt like a mini-ICU instead of a farmhouse. He now had a feeding tube and a colostomy bag. The caregivers were thorough and always asked for guidance or alerted me if they noted any changes in the patient's condition they were caring for. I would go out and assess the situation as needed. I was also in regular contact with their primary care provider as part of this health care team, to collaborate on their behalf.

Having care in the home and all the ancillary resources that were available to them helped facilitate this existence. We pulled in community resources whenever it was necessary to help make this situation feasible.

Mr. C passed away comfortably at home listening to his favorite songs on the radio early one morning, surrounded by his wife, family, and trusted caregivers. It was a peaceful passing, and unfortunately, hospice was not involved to make the transition smoother. While Mrs. C was very sad to lose her partner of sixty-five years, she grew to accept the loss but looked fondly back at the many memories they had together, including aging in place. After her husband's passing, we were able to have a psychotherapist come talk to her for the next six months and she had therapy in the home on a regular basis, which helped her cope with her loss and other issues in her life. The family found these sessions especially helpful, as their mother was getting the help she needed right at home.

A year later, Mrs. C had a stroke and was unable to communicate due to loss of speech. Again, the family opted to have all options made available to keep her alive. She remained a full code at the family's insistence. While in the rehabilitation center after her stroke, our caregivers were providing private duty care to her when one of them witnessed an event that she reported to the son. The caregiver stepped in to advocate for Mrs. C as she was unable to do so for herself, and the family was very appreciative. The facility's employee was very rough on Mrs. C while administering care one day and spoke curtly to her. Mrs. C became fearful of this employee; she did not have the ability to articulate her feelings, but whenever this employee would appear, her eyes would grow wide with fear and trepidation as she recalled the episode where she felt vulnerable and helpless. She relied heavily on her private duty caregiver to be there for her and assist her with all of her physical needs that she could not communicate. Her caregiver became her communicator and protector because she knew her needs so well.

Her private duty caregiver came into her shift one evening and witnessed Mrs. C holding a glass of water in her hand resting on her lap as she was dozing off in bed. The caregiver was upset at seeing this, as she knew that Mrs. C was ordered to have nothing by mouth due to her inability to safely swallow after her stroke (dysphagia). By not following orders, the staff had again put Mrs. C in harm's way. This was an unintentional outcome, as the employees in a health care setting are extremely busy and usually understaffed, which elevates the potential for danger to those most in need of care. The private caregiver provided vital added assistance for Mrs. C and made her feel comfortable and safe.

The family soon realized that Mrs. C really wanted to be in the comfort of her own home and requested discharge. We worked with the facility to facilitate this as soon as they found it safe to do so. We had Mrs. C discharged home to live out the remainder of her life where she felt the most comfortable. We have been told by administrators through the years that it does not seem safe for patients with high-acuity needs to be capably cared for in their homes; however, we have been able to provide a high level of patient care in conjunction with making a variety of resources available to families right in their own homes. Patients in these situations have been among our most satisfied clients.

Outcome:

Mrs. C eventually passed away in the hospital. The family again wanted every measure taken to try to save her, but despite all efforts, she passed away. With every hospital stay, there is debilitation and physical decline. In my experience, each day one lies in a hospital bed; it necessitates about three days recovering. Therefore, successive hospital stays create a cumulative negative effect on the body which can overwhelm and eventually lead to the weakening of the various bodily systems, especially in elderly patients. While the family was deeply saddened, they felt comfortable that there was no unfinished business, as their parents' wishes were obeyed until their last breaths.

In the end, the family had no regrets for either of their parents. The children were satisfied that their parents received the best care possible, and they were satisfied with the fact that they were able to maximize their years the best they could.

A serendipitous outcome of our care for this couple was that the family became the source of many referrals for our business and became an extension of our family. They were one of our first clients and helped us develop strategies to care not only for them but for all future patients as well.

Advocacy tips :

The major difference with this advocacy case was that the family wanted "everything done to keep their parents alive." This is not a typical request, but for this family it was, and our goal was to honor their wishes. During hospital or ER stays, even the hospitalists would try and explain to the family that heroic measures can be detrimental to the outcome of patients; the family truly did not want to hear it. This was a lovely family, and they are entitled to a plan where they are all in agreement. While my personal feelings may differ from theirs, the important part of being a supportive advocate is to support the family and not project my own feelings onto them or to try to convince them that I am right and they are wrong. We did well together.

- When caring for the elderly, you want to advocate for and focus on comfort measures, nutrition for strength, skin breakdown prevention, infection control to minimize infections and cross contamination between the two. In doing so, identify the goal, and then outline your approach to meet the goal with a measurable outcome to monitor if you met your goals .
- Tap into community resources when needed to optimize care at home. The best part about the Cs is that they could live out their lives in their own home rather than live in a facility, which was always their desire. They remained at home with frequent visits from their children and grandchildren, which always brought a smile to their faces. Even their neighbors were supportive and came to know the family caregivers over the years.
- When caring for the elderly at home who need frequent ER trips, you need to ensure that they have coverage and become familiar with their doctors so you can coordinate their medication management and appointments.

· Chapter 6 ·

Difficult Dementia

"When we are no longer able to change a situation, we are challenged to change ourselves."

—Viktor Frankl

We met Sam when he was sixty-five years young and had been suffering from Lewy body dementia (LBD) for six years. He and his wife lived in a beautiful home in the suburbs. His career as a physician had ended abruptly due to his illness, but his wife continued to work and had a thriving career, which is why she needed help with her husband. Since he was the third generation to present with dementia in his family, he was not a stranger to this disease and this was a very sensitive topic for his family.

When we met Sam, he was having problems with walking, feeding himself, communication, mood swings, and depression, and did not recognize his children. Sam had other comorbidities as well, including osteoporosis, high cholesterol, anxiety, depression, and hypothyroidism. He had lost twenty-five pounds in the past couple of years and his wife's emotional "tank" was getting low. On assessment day, I suggested moving him to the first floor for his safety, but the family was resistant to this change initially.

> LBD was discovered by Dr. Friederich Lewy in the early 1900s when he was researching Parkinson's disease. He discovered these abnormal protein deposits in the brain that disrupt brain function, which he called Lewy body proteins. LBD can present as early as fifty years old. It is progressive. Although it leads to a decline in thinking, reasoning, and independence as it relates to all activities of living, each individual with LBD will experience the symptoms of dementia differently. The disease may cause a wide range of symptoms, including memory loss, changes in alertness and attention, sleep issues, visual hallucinations, problems with movement and posture, muscle stiffness, and confusion.

Because Sam could not communicate his thoughts and because others were not able to understand him, he was understandably and visibly frustrated. He had a level of awareness that something was not right with him. To us, he looked like a healthy sixty-year-old man, but when he attempted to communicate, it was apparent that he was not. He lived day to day seemingly trapped in a web that walled him off from the world of communication as we know it. His frustration led him to be combative and seemingly uncooperative to his caregivers and family when they tried to help him. This aggression was not willful and was due to Sam not comprehending why people were touching him or doing things to him that he used to do himself without thinking, such as bathing, wiping himself, feeding himself, and all activities of daily living that we do without thought when we are well and able.

Awareness is pivotal in dealing with a person like Sam; it is vital to be aware of their ability to swing or act out at any moment and to understand that they are acting out in response to their confusion related to their disease process. Along with this awareness, it is important to speak to them in the same manner you would a person who can fully understand and communicate. Speak to them as if they understand each action you are about to take. This is done because there are moments of clarity in this disease process, and dignity for each person is the standard by which we treat others. Surprise moves without explanation are more apt to cause a person with dementia to "act out" with aggression. It is much more effective to explain a task and to move slowly while working with them. For example, when a caregiver is attempting to remove a patient's clothing without verbal warning, this can trigger a response that could include being combative. Instead, if you speak clearly and slowly about each action that will transpire, you can potentially reduce aggression. Caregivers are instructed to move slowly and inform the patient, in a calm reassuring voice, of each and every move they will make.

Sam also had an unsteady gait related to his shuffling, another symptom related to LBD. This gait presented a fall risk, and ascending or descending the stairs became tricky for him. We orchestrated a plan whereby he went down the stairs once in the morning after morning care, and he did not go back upstairs until bedtime. He was a fall risk not just for himself but also for his spouse and his caregiver who assisted him, especially when navigating the stairs. Before this care plan went into effect there were several near misses which made implementing the plan even more important for everyone's safety.

A customized care plan was written and reviewed with the caregivers and Sam's wife to keep everyone on the same page. LBD was discussed at length with the caregivers so they could be familiar with some of the issues that Sam was facing and be empathetic to his needs while keeping him safe. The identified issues included safety/fall risk, risk of dehydration, proper nutrition, tracking elimination patterns, appropriate exercise routines, and brain stimulation with conversations or activities that kept Sam occupied or interested as much as possible. Sam was also being seen by a primary care provider as well as a geriatric psychiatrist to help manage some of his behaviors and mood.

Because of all this, Sam was unable to be left alone. Nights became difficult because Sam did not always want to sleep at the same time as his wife. Wandering around at the top of a large staircase was a risk, and soon his spouse felt that she had to sleep with one eye open. Caregiver stress takes its toll on a spouse and lack of sleep contributes to this stress. Adding a night caregiver is typically the last option before a family needs to make alternative decisions about safe placement when it becomes too much for the family to handle.

For eleven months, we were able to work with Sam in his home and provide care that met his needs as well as his family's needs safely. And then I began getting messages from the caregivers that safety on the stairs was becoming a bigger issue, so after a few close calls, I felt we needed to address the issue. His wife tried to keep any safety concerns that she was having a secret. She felt like she was failing as a spouse/caregiver to admit that the situation was becoming overwhelming. She also wanted to protect her children from this pain; some were married with kids, but they had a younger child still in high school.

After meeting with Sam's caregivers to collect information and the specifics of their concerns about the safety of Sam in his home, I put together a list of concerns that identified where Sam was at risk for safety, comfort, and quality of life. I then invited a clinical social worker that I often work with and the family to my office for a meeting to help address the psychosocial issues that come with a discussion like this.

At the meeting, I presented them with my concerns and the clinical social worker addressed some of their difficult emotions; we had a very informative and successful meeting. In the end, the family decided to place their father in an alternate living situation that they all felt comfortable with. I gave them several places to visit to see what "felt" right for their father. In the next several weeks, they visited these different places and they decided to move Sam to a small, eight-person group home. They utilized Sam's caregivers in the transition due to their familiarity, and Sam settled in nicely over the next couple of months. They were able to select a group home that felt like a "home" and were told that they could keep their father there until the end of his life. This was very important as the thought of additional moves in the future is very stressful, especially with a dementia patient. Minimizing insults is always the best option.

Outcome:

Sam lived another two years, and the family did well with his transition into a small group home. All of his mental, physical, and emotional needs were met until his last breath. The family felt that their father's care left no stone unturned. While difficult for all of them, they felt that Sam's last years yielded satisfaction on every front and gave them peace of mind. They could visit him as often as they wanted, and the group home was able to assume the role of his family doing all his personal care, keeping him safe, and ensuring he was very well cared for. Sam's wife continues to work full time and enjoy life with their family while living a full and active life, which was critical to her as she is only in her sixties and has yet to retire.

Advocacy tips:

Dementia in a loved one is a difficult disorder for families to deal with, especially early-onset dementia. I deal with dementia patients and their families on a daily basis.

- When helping a family cope with their loved one's dementia, it is important to help them understand that dementia causes unintentional behaviors. In essence, the patients' oppositional behavior is not willful; they do not intentionally act difficult. A person with dementia is very much in the moment and that moment can look very different from one minute to the next. These circumstances and behaviors are all disease related.

- When caring for the patient, it is important to watch out for frustration and depression as they are aware on some level that things are not quite right with them, and things they used to do without even thinking about do not come easily. They struggle for words, they struggle to use the remote control, and they can't operate the phone or even know how to turn on a light switch. Many times these are highly intelligent people with bright minds who held very high-level professional careers. When they do have a lucid moment, the reality of their situation can come rushing in and their awareness leads to anger, but the moment is so fleeting that they soon lose that moment of awareness. Dementia is not just memory impairment but can also affect the executive functioning portion of the brain to include working memory, flexible thinking, insight, judgement, and self-control.

- Since there are generally five main diseases that cause dementia (Alzheimer's disease, LBD, Vascular Dementia, Frontotemporal Dementia, and Mixed Dementia) and other medical conditions that can appear to have the same symptoms as dementia but have very different causes (Huntington's disease, normal pressure hydrocephalus, Parkinson's disease, traumatic brain injury, Creutzfeldt-Jakob disease, and Wernicke-Korsakoff Syndrome), it is important to ensure the medical provider does a complete medical and neurological workup before assuming what their medical condition is. Workups should include labs, scans, and a complete physical examination by a licensed medical provider. Medications should be reviewed to make sure they are not contributing to the cognitive decline of an individual. Medical history should include a history of head injury or trauma and timelines should be reviewed carefully in conjunction with the timing of when symptoms first began.

Some helpful tips I offer to families of dementia patients:

- Do not shame your loved one if they repeat the same question or statement over and over and you constantly remind them that they have done this. You can contribute to their increased anxiety, frustration, and depression, which, in turn, causes their cognition to be worse.
- Don't correct them unless they ask you to clarify a date or a statement. Don't tell them "you keep saying that."
- Don't tell them "you're wrong." Just go with what they say. One tenet I live by is that it is more important to be kind than to be right.
- Distract your loved one if they seem to be perseverating on a topic. "I really like that outfit you have on; is it new? How is your son? What is the dog's name? Let's look at this book right here."
- Don't remind them repeatedly that someone they cared about passed away. If they ask where a person who passed away is, you can let this lead to another topic about that person's life. You can certainly be honest with them, but you will find that if they keep asking the same question, that each time they hear the news they will respond as if it is the first time and will cause much anguish over and over. This is painful and traumatic, which is why the distraction is helpful. You can change the subject or ask them what their favorite pastime was with that person.

- Be patient, respectful, and always be polite. We recently had a woman ask where her deceased husband was, which she did up to twenty times per day, and the caregiver decided to say he was playing golf, one of his favorite pastimes. As the wife looked out the window, she said, "It is getting dark; he should be home soon." She then easily went onto another topic.

- Don't give too many choices or open-ended questions like, "What do you want for breakfast?" Instead offer two choices only: "Do you want cereal or pancakes?" Open-ended questions are confusing because they cannot recall their options.

- When telling them about what you plan on doing with them, only give them one command at a time. "Let's get your shoes on. Let's take a ride." If you tell them you are going to get their shoes on, go for a ride, and go to the store, they lose their ability to track what you just said as they become more confused. It is an overload of information. Their brain does not work like it used to.

- Talk to them like the adult that they are, not like they are a child. They sense this and feel like they are being treated in a condescending way.

- Don't talk about a person in front of them. Despite having dementia, they can still hear and should be respected as adults. They are able to feel shame, sadness, and anger.

- Don't laugh at them; laugh with them. Sometimes they know they mixed something up and laugh at it. It is OK to do that, but to laugh at them is shaming them when they say something inaccurately.
- Don't tell your loved one that they are going to an appointment the next morning and expect them to remember it when they wake up. Also, this little bit of information can stress them and keep them awake even if they don't recall what they were told. New information, appointments, and company coming can all cause an uneasiness that can set them off, but they cannot articulate this uneasiness. They can't recall very well and even written notes are not always the answer.

All of these tips are much easier said than done, but the answer is patience and kindness. This advice seems so simple, yet it is hard when it is your loved one who is so repetitive that it is taxing to be in their presence for too long. It is OK to step outside and collect yourself; this is a very difficult disease on many levels.

I understand because I have faced it myself. Again, in the rearview mirror, we are going for no regrets. If after a loved one passes away, we are burdened by how we treated them, then this is difficult to resolve. Having assistance to deal with them in the present is the way to go to get you to feeling at peace when they have left you.

· Chapter 7 ·

First Surgery at Eighty

"There is a calmness to a life lived in gratitude, a quiet joy."

—Ralph H. Blum

Pain will get your attention, especially if you are eighty years old, have never had pain in your life, and suddenly have pain all day and night with no good explanation. In other words, you did not engage in any new activity or exercises that would have caused your pain, but now it plagues you.

This is what happened to Delores in 2008. As an eighty-year-old woman who lived on her own, she was very active. She had a stair climber mobility chair in place for her husband since 2000 and simply kept it in the home after he passed away in 2003. She was able to do all her own chores, laundry, meals, and yardwork up until this time. She could not drive so she took Metro-Access for all pre-scheduled events. If last-minute rides were needed, she would call her family or close friends, who never minded being her chauffeur. She was still active in her church group, garden club, and was continuously busy with her large and growing extended family. Life was good for her and her favorite comment had always been, "I love life!" It showed in her effervescent ways. Each night she would express gratitude for the ability to enjoy the day, and she truly did enjoy each and every single day.

Even in her declining health, her life was full of joy. Her life had always been full of joy. She was raised in a small town in northwest Pennsylvania, then traveled to Philadelphia to become a nurse. Initially, she worked in the operating room as a circulating nurse in the 1950s. After meeting her husband, they started a family, and she took a thirty-year hiatus to travel the world and raise her five children. Their travels took them from Pennsylvania to Europe for four years, where they lived in France and Germany while her husband worked on military contracts for IBM. They traveled by cruise liner in 1964 from New York City with their four young children as their parents and extended family watched from the harbor. This was an almost unheard of venture in the 1960s, but off they went. In 1968, they returned to the United States, again by cruise liner, with now five children in tow. Delores and her family settled this time in the suburbs of Washington, DC, where they have been since. In fact, Delores remained in the home they purchased that year, a desire she was very verbal about in 2008 when she developed this acute pain in her left hip.

In 1980, Delores returned to her nursing career at a local nursing home, where she soon fell in love with caring for the elderly residents. She returned to work part time, renewing her nursing license after almost thirty years, when her fourth child graduated high school. But in 2004, when she lost her vision, her nursing career came to an abrupt halt. She had taken her grandchildren to a park with some friends from her hometown of Ridgway, Pennsylvania, but could not drive home due to her sudden loss of central vision. As it turned out, she developed what is called a macular hemorrhage in both eyes, very suddenly without explanation, and was deemed legally blind from this point on. She had been diagnosed with macular degeneration seven years prior, but it was being monitored every six months by an ophthalmologist, and did not require treatment up until this time.

Her sudden vision loss led to my becoming her advocate, fueling my passion for this career that has continued to this day. We saw a retina specialist who told her that she met the criteria of being legally blind because her visual acuity was less than 20/200 in her best eye. I will never forget this day because Delores asked her doctor what this meant for her, and his response was, "You will figure it out." Delores was stymied by his answer, as was I. We were given no resources or pamphlets or places to call. As her advocate, it became my job to figure out how to best allow Delores to live a quality life with her current situation. The doctor also said, "You obviously can't drive." And with those words, her career as a geriatric nurse ended, but as she typically did, she chose the high road and her life became filled with adventure, optimism, and hope.

This was where her community also came into play. Her neighbor, Sharon, suggested we call her mother, who eventually helped us formulate a plan for how to live with this newly acquired impairment. Through the Jewish Social Services Agency (JSSA), we made contact with an agency for the visually impaired and a consultation was set up. I was connected with a blind woman who came out to the house and spent a day with Delores to help her "feel her way around" and mark on/off switches, mark alarm clocks, and mark the oven, all with raised dots that would help Delores feel her way. After this woman left for the day, Delores felt empowered. She told me if a woman can live alone with no sight and only a white cane, she certainly can figure this out with 20/200 sight. She planned a dinner party for the following week and made it happen. After her dinner party, Delores never looked back. She moved on and sold her car, accepting her new life and verbalizing how grateful she was to still be able to hear, stay in her home, and just figure it all out. It was the first of many dinner parties for Delores, and her life moved on. Though sometimes food was a bit too salty or the baking soda was mismeasured, it did not matter; she remained independent and optimistic. We were able to get her set up with Metro-Access, we hired Clara to pay her bills, and life was looking pretty bright despite Delores's newfound "darkness." She continued to focus on all the good that life had given her, counted every blessing she had, and still continued to help others at every turn.

In 2008, *Nursing Spectrum*, a national nursing publication, nominated Delores as runner-up for Nurse of the Year in the Washington, DC, metropolitan area after several neighbors and acquaintances wrote letters to support why she was deserving of such an award. I attended the banquet with her at the Four Seasons Hotel and was in awe of such a lady. Her favorite line was "I love life!" She prepared a speech about how much she enjoyed her life and her career "in white." Speaking to all the young nurses, she described how much nursing had changed since the day she graduated in 1949 and said she would never change a thing; her life experiences had shaped and molded her.

Other than her visual issues, she had only been diagnosed with one condition her whole life, monoclonal gammopathy of undetermined significance (MGUS) which was being monitored carefully by her hematologist. This condition was found during a routine blood workup in the early 1980s, and did require a bone marrow biopsy, which proved to be negative. Simply put, the body creates an abnormal protein and it needs monitoring because when an individual has this condition, it puts them at increased risk of developing bone marrow and blood diseases. Routine blood work was done annually, and this was never a problem, but in 2008, with this new complaint of excruciating pain in her left hip, the suspicion of a bone marrow disease resurfaced. I kept copies of all her labs to show the detailed history of her MGUS.

We visited her orthopedist. Though multiple scans were done, no good explanation was found. Her pain continued, and nothing seemed to alleviate the pain as she became more immobile each day. She had Clara help do her household chores a few days a week, as she was not able to do much on her own. We decided she should get a second opinion from another orthopedist to try and figure out this pain. He ordered more tests and another MRI was done. Interestingly, each physician has radiological centers that they prefer so you can end up having multiple MRIs, which seems redundant but is protocol. About ten days after the tests were ordered, we were told to come back and do a follow-up visit. Delores was now in a wheelchair due to the pain and her immobility. This was the strangest appointment I had ever attended in my life. The doctor seemed disorganized and the computers "were down," so he could not access the scans, but he told us that it appeared that Delores had bone disease, most likely cancer, which was causing her pain, and to go home and get her "affairs in order." I queried him about what to do next as

Delores's advocate, and he told me that I could either "take the bumpy path outside his office and wheel her over to the local hospital or better yet drive five miles away" where there was an orthopedic oncologist who could help address her seemingly terminal diagnosis. To say we were blown away is truly an understatement. Just like that, we were facing Delores's mortality and her "time to get her affairs in order." Again, Delores took the high road. A woman of faith and conviction, she said, "It will be OK."

As her advocate and at a total loss for what to do next, I crossed the parking lot to get the car. As I was walking, a woman named Sue from the radiology center next door saw my face and asked me what was wrong. Being a nurse practitioner, Sue happened to recognize me from working in the building upstairs and knew that Delores had had a scan at her office the week before. Sue told me that the computers were down, but that the information we had been given did not sound right to her, and she went to go get me a copy of the actual report. Talk about divine intervention: the timing of my meeting her in the parking lot and her reading the dismay on my face, then intervening when she did, was truly unbelievable. She came out with a report that did not reveal what the doctor had just told us. The report showed an abnormality in her femur that was possibly from avascular necrosis (AVN) but no mention of cancer was noted in the report anywhere. I was literally scratching my head, as this was not a life-threatening condition. I did not know which way to turn. At the time, I was working part-time in two practices, a Gastroenterology (GI) practice and a complex integrative medical practice. I called the physician at the latter and told him what was going on. I told him Delores had a pain level of 10/10; it was a Thursday evening around 6 p.m., and I simply did not know which direction to turn. Again, I felt such relief when my boss said, "Bring Delores here, and we will give her some fluids and see if we can't get her some pain relief in our infusion center." This intervention temporarily helped Delores with some pain relief. However, the news we had been given two hours earlier to get her affairs in order had prompted a phone call to her entire family of over twenty people, who were waiting in her living room when I brought Delores home. Tears of anguish, confusion, and shock greeted us when we got her home at nearly 9 p.m. I needed to figure out how I could best help Delores in this still unclear medical crisis. We would come up with a plan in the morning, but emotions were high. Delores's pain was a bit better since her IVs, but I had no idea what was going on, as what the doctor said and what the MRI report stated were vastly different. We got Delores settled into bed, one of her sons stayed with her, and I told her I would be back in the morning to drive her to the hospital. Lost and confused does not begin to describe what had just transpired over the previous six hours. Yet through it all, Delores remained optimistic and comforted her family by telling them that whatever happened, it would all work out. I was not so sure and felt like I was with Delores on a roller coaster. But sometimes there are plans bigger than us, and we simply are not aware of how mumbled prayers are being answered.

Amy was working that day in the ER; she is the most gracious and helpful ER nurse I have ever met. Amy always helps "get it done!" Amazing, truly amazing! With all that, I had a glimmer of hope I had not felt in twenty-four hours since finding out that Delores seemingly was facing her final challenge in life. Again, divine intervention felt like it showed up when Dr. O came to the bedside and asked what was going on with Delores. I told him the information Delores's second-opinion physician had given us, and he said, "OK, we will handle this, but best-case scenario, she will have a hip replacement and be on her way in a week!" I was a bit skeptical, as I was still hearing the conversation from the previous afternoon telling us to get Delores's affairs in order. Within two hours, we had seen Delores's hematologist who felt that her labs did not reflect that of multiple myeloma (a bone marrow cancer disorder associated with MGUS), and yet another MRI was done. The final verdict was avascular necrosis, also known as AVN, the death of bone tissue due to a lack of blood supply, which is very, very painful and explained Delores's recent pain. She had one "hole" in the bone, and Dr. O felt pretty strongly that this was not cancerous at all, but the surgery would be the gold standard of diagnosing exactly what was going on.

Within forty-eight hours, Delores had surgery on her left hip and her immediate future looked much brighter than the previous fifty-two hours. There was NO cancer, the pain had all stemmed from this AVN, and she sailed through the surgery with flying colors. Delores's situation went from hopeless to quite bright in the course of a few days, thanks to guidance and direction from a friend who showed up at the right time, a physician we trusted, and a sound plan.

During this hospitalization, Delores developed low sodium levels in her blood, known as hyponatremia, and a workup was done that confirmed she had Addison's disease. Addison's disease is a disorder of the adrenal glands where they don't produce enough hormones, specifically cortisol. Delores was put on treatment for this by a nephrologist and stabilized. Her sodium level came back to normal, and she was now on a low dose of steroids daily.

After what started off as a harrowing experience but turned into a completely manageable and tolerable situation, Delores, now pain free and fully ambulatory, went home with physical therapy and a new lease on life.

Outcome:

As an advocate, this was one of my most frustrating cases. But the outcome was so good that we wasted little emotion on being told completely wrong information. We chose to celebrate the new lease on life and not look back. To this day, I have contemplated what the doctor who told Delores to get her affairs in order would do if we walked in to see him twelve years after the fact?

The community, in this case, also helped guide us. I was extremely grateful that Janet called when she did, that she went out on a limb to contact Dr. O, and that Dr. O was so willing to help us. He is a phenomenal doctor and has been involved in many lifesaving procedures with some acquaintances of mine, and again, I feel such gratitude to those medical professionals who have always helped me along the way in navigating difficult situations.

Advocacy tips:

- Always search for answers and don't give up. Sometimes it helps to take a step back first and think before acting. In this case, I reached out to my boss, Dr. F, at a difficult time to help Delores get some temporary relief until we could come up with a game plan in the morning. Even Delores herself had asked us to let her sleep on it and start fresh in the morning to seek clarity for her situation.
- Remain calm and be pragmatic while looking for answers. And don't forget to turn to your community as needed.
- Be aware that often when a patient goes in for treatment of one condition, another one surfaces, as was the case with Delores's hyponatremia. Thankfully, we were able to get that under control with the help of an outstanding nephrologist and her primary care doctor, who remained involved throughout the whole process.

· Chapter 8 ·

Please, Help Me

"Be the witness of your thoughts. You are what observes, not what you observe."

—Buddhist proverb

In December 2010, I received a call from a gentleman in DC. He had obtained my name through an owner of a family-owned pharmacy in the District of Columbia, who had gotten my name from Becky, the owner of a chain of small group homes. Six months prior, I had reached out to her on behalf of a client who needed immediate placement, and she had helped facilitate this with great success. The small-group-home option was a very good fit for my client, and it also introduced me to the world and advantages of small group homes in the Washington, DC, metropolitan area. Becky told the pharmacy owner he should call me and see if I could help his friend Jeffrey.

Jeffrey, a sixty-five-year-old gentleman in a wheelchair, had taken ill in August and was in a difficult mental and physical state. He was overwhelmed and not sure what to do next to get his life "back on track." He had a very reliable sister who had helped him make all the decisions to this point, but she really needed help as she was juggling a career, family, and a sick brother all at the same time.

We met a few days before Christmas at his lovely home on Capitol Hill. He had suddenly found himself feeble and not able to take care of himself. He was very frustrated after multiple prolonged and frequent hospital and rehabilitation stays. He told me that while he was certain that the medical care that brought him to this place was less than optimal, he did not want to rehash it in a litigious arena; he just wanted to get better and move on. He said his goals were to gain independence, avoid further complications, eradicate pain, obtain a "healthy" mental state, walk independently, and once again, travel the world and work independently as he did prior to this illness.

Unfortunately, he had contracted a terrible infection in multiple joints after multiple epidural injections. This led to sepsis (infection in the bloodstream), multiple protracted courses of antibiotics, and the inability to ambulate independently. His current health issues included the inability to ambulate safely on his own without a walker, urinary issues, anxiety, weight gain from prolonged inactivity, chronic pain, opioid dependence, and complete dependence on caregivers for all of his activities of daily living.

Initially, when he met with me, he was hesitant to engage my services, as he wanted a physician versus a nurse practitioner. I told him that was certainly understandable, and I would send him a care plan, then he could get back to me when he decided what he wanted to do.

He accepted my care plan, signed appropriate documents ensuring confidentiality, and our journey began. Over the next six years, I assumed the role of his health advocate, and when I would go to a doctor's appointment with him and the doctor would ask my role, Jeffrey would jokingly quip, "She is my bodyguard." While initially my appearance with Jeffrey seemed to make some medical providers uneasy, they soon understood that my position was simply to help Jeffrey navigate his new complex medical journey. I went to each appointment with a binder full of his medical information, including procedures, lab results, diagnostic test results, discharge summaries from each hospital stay, medical diagnoses, and treating physician information. This ensured he and the doctors had no confusion about the details of his difficult medical journey and his visits were never disjointed due to holes in his treatment records. His clinical picture and timeline were always clear at each visit. I was able to establish a rapport with Jeffrey's providers to the point that they would take texts from me or call me for clarification. I functioned as the hub on his wheel supporting all the spokes as I coordinated his care from every level. Jeffrey trusted me, and we began his journey to health and recovery. Jeffrey felt that due to his pain medications and dimmed mental state, he would not have been able to retain the information that I collected at each appointment, and we established a relationship of trust and transparency. I would then facilitate getting the updated information to his medical care team as well as his sister. Medication prescriptions were filled, pill boxes were changed, and his care plan was continuously updated to keep everyone on his team abreast of changes.

Jeffrey had caregivers in his home that helped him one-on-one and knew the best way to help him. Each caregiver was carefully selected and trained to help move him along the continuum to his health goals. He was open to them being present for him even when he started to feel better and felt perhaps they weren't needed, but because he never wanted to end up worse, he always erred on the side of caution.

One issue in this business is cutting back caregivers' hours before the client is actually ready to do so, and then suffering the consequences of this action. We often try to explain that cutting from eight hours to zero hours is a bad idea. Instead, it is better to gradually reduce the hours to ensure the safety and well-being of the patient, averting preventable issues such as falls. Jeffrey was never in the hospital or rehab alone; we always kept a well-trained caregiver with him to avoid any potential pitfalls that would cause him to backslide in his progress. Some nights I was up all night with him in the hospital and would not leave until another team member was with him and he was "settled," be that in the hospital or back home. Communication was pivotal to all team members as to what was happening with Jeffrey, and any change in plans had to be communicated so they could be at the right place to care for him. I always spoke with the doctors in the hospital, relayed information to his family, and then followed up with changing his care plan to reflect the most current "snapshot" of his health. This is a continual process, but when done pragmatically, it helps the patient progress with the best outcome. The team approach was the only way to be on the same page with one another. We became very adept at communicating any concerns, questions, or changes through the chain, and then I would reach out to his medical provider for answers which facilitated his positive outcome. We were able to keep the caregivers on board with the continually updated plan of care and each step of Jeffrey's day was reviewed with them in the form of a "to-do list." It was a team approach. Occasionally, we had to remove a caregiver if they were not a good fit, but our communication patterns were always clear and Jeffrey's best interest was always our focus. He also provided frequent feedback in this area, as he was the one being cared for, so if he felt an individual was not a good fit, we listened to him.

I attended each emergency room visit, every doctor's appointment, and every surgery or procedure that Jeffrey had. We met monthly to review and update goals and stay current with all his medical issues. Along the way, we involved the additional services of licensed professionals: dieticians, LCSWs, physical therapists, RNs, and even an acupuncturist. When Jeffrey began traveling initially, he was accompanied by caregivers. From December 2010 through December 2016, I attended hundreds of visits with him.

In 2012, Jeffrey underwent knee replacement surgery with a specialist in Virginia who specialized in infections in joints. He was terrified to have surgery after all he had been through, but he was having problems walking, and this was affecting his quality of life once again. After we met this specialist from a highly regarded clinic, Jeffrey and I felt like it was a good fit as his specialty was so specific. He was very aware of how to prepare Jeffrey for surgery in the safest way possible to prevent him from getting another MRSA infection, like he had when he was initially sick. He worked with Jeffrey and me over the course of six months until he felt like it was safe for him to have his knee replacement without an increased risk of infection. Jeffrey did great with this surgery and never had any post-operative complications to this day.

In 2017, his goals were met and he was once again traveling independently throughout the world to promote business development in underdeveloped countries as a consultant, which he had been doing for the past twenty-seven years. Once he was well enough to travel abroad, we discussed that if there were an emergency, I would fly to him and pick up the advocacy responsibilities in whichever country he happened to be in. We were determined to get him to the "finish line" the best we could. At that point, we only met face to face once a year as an annual follow-up.

Even though I was working full time at another job while doing Jeffrey's advocacy, I never missed work as, interestingly enough, he typically only had emergencies arise in the evening after work or during the night. I also trained and hired some nurses who understood advocacy to accompany Jeffrey when I was not available, and this was fine with him as well.

He met his goals, he surpassed his goals, and he was open to every approach to make this happen.

Outcome:

In Jeffrey's own words: *In August 2010, I became very ill with an infectious disease. I was hospitalized, then sent to rehab, and then hospitalized again.*

My sibling was my advocate and spared no effort to try to help me. However, neither she nor I were familiar with either the intricacies of the medical system or [the] complex medical technology.

I observed that the hospitals, the rehab center, and the insurance providers all had "case managers." But they were managing the "case" from their perspective—not mine.

I asked around if there were a way for me to have a case manager. About four months after my original illness, I was introduced to Andrea Kohn. My sister and I met with her. I engaged her.

For the next two years, I was hospitalized and back in rehab a number of times. My mind was often foggy, and I was often depressed from the medication.

Andrea managed my case in an outstanding manner. I managed to largely stay at home as opposed to a facility. For many months, I had twenty-four-hour, in-home aides who were supervised and coordinated by Andrea. Over time this was reduced from sixteen hours to twelve hours, then six hours, and then zero. Andrea guided that process, including particularly knowing when reductions could be made, and in one situation where it had to be increased. This was a two-year process.

I had a strong desire to not go into the hospital or rehab unnecessarily. On a number of occasions, Andrea coordinated to bring health care professionals to my home for things for which I would have otherwise had no choice but to go to the hospital.

On the one occasion when hospitalization was necessary, Andrea made the judgement. I was taken by ambulance to the hospital and was in emergency and intensive care for a number of days. Andrea was with me for the first fifteen or more hours. She had all of my records and an intimate knowledge of my medical history. At a minimum, the result was that I needed many fewer tests, and at most, I would not have otherwise survived. When I wanted to leave the hospital, she arranged, against the will of the hospital, to get me into rehab and home.

I had a new infection and my home needed to be "decontaminated" and she coordinated that.

Over a period of about three years, she went with me to doctor's and other medical appointments. Because of the medication, I was only sometimes able to be fully attentive. I never had full grasp of the medical terminology. She was able to communicate with the doctors, ask the correct questions, give informed answers to their questions, and then help me make sometimes complex decisions. I believe the result was that I had fewer surgeries and procedures than I would have otherwise have had.

Over the following eighteen months, when my condition was no longer life- threatening, she coordinated my medical care, including arranging for aides when I traveled.

Over the six years since she has continued to periodically check in with me, maintain my medical records, and on a few occasions, when I requested, come to medical appointments with me.

His family was so grateful for his success and that they could continue to enjoy their brother, uncle, and cousin. I only see Jeffrey typically once a year now, and he has remained very healthy and met his goal of traveling the world and got back to his consulting position in 2017. He has been one of my biggest referral networks, and he taught me much. He continues to touch base with me from some of the most remote parts of the world, and it is always nice to hear from him. I am still privy to his annual physical examination reports, and he contacts me when he is in need of any medical advice.

Advocacy tips:

Jeffrey's case highlights a hands-on approach to advocacy in a very complex patient where my nurse practitioner education served me well. He required quite a bit of care, guidance, and time. But by working with him, I learned to trust in myself and to always ask questions.

- It helps when the patient is open to every aspect of the caregiver's suggestions, as Jeffrey was. As an advocate, you want to make sure you gain their trust and that they value your opinion. To do this, research the best providers and ensure your patient always feels comfortable with each specialist.
- Your success should be based on their success. So, make sure to plan meetings to continually stay in contact, discuss particulars, and then tweak anything that does not seem to be working. This case became a fine-tuned machine and helped us to establish procedures for other clients who needed health advocacy.
- You want to micromanage your patient's health care to prevent many issues that could delay their progress.
- When you work with a team of caregivers, make sure that each and every caregiver plays a very special role in their work with the patient. Ensure that every caregiver becomes adept at noticing if urine

has an odor or if a sore is developing or if diarrhea seems infectious rather than a virus. Let them know they can contact you and ask any questions.

· Chapter 9 ·

Two Hours, and Then You'll Be Home

"Calmness is a huge gift. And once you master it, you will be able to respond in a useful way to every difficult situation that decides to walk into your heart."

—Geri Larkin

On May 11th, 2014, Delores boarded a plane for Atlanta, Georgia, for her grandson's college graduation. At this point, she was eighty-six years young, and other than her legal blindness due to macular degeneration (chapter 7), she was getting along quite well. Her one and only surgery was her hip replacement six years prior.

With her great attitude, she was able to attend the commencement weekend. She enjoyed her grandson's graduation, a couple of special meals, and the next day, she flew back to Maryland with her family. It was a special three days for the family.

We were very careful with Delores while in Atlanta. With Delores's limited sight, someone needed to help her safely navigate unfamiliar surroundings. Sidewalks, uneven carpets, throw rugs, and many uneven surfaces present challenges to the visibly impaired. Delores has never been one to complain even when her vision was 20/400 and worsening each year.

The following Sunday after graduation, Delores went to church with family as she typically did, and on the way in that morning, her heel caught the rubber mat by the door. Luckily, a very attentive usher caught sight of this and actually caught her before she hit the ground. She seemed OK and went on about her business that day.

All seemed well, but in the following days and weeks, she began to experience pain in her left hip and lower back area.

Over the course of the next two months, we would see two orthopedists and have several MRIs and comprehensive workups without a clear definition of why Delores remained in pain. This was similar to her issues in chapter

7. The MRI scans indicated that during her fall, she tore muscles and tendons in her hip and pelvic region, and these take time to repair. She began physical therapy but had to cut it short as she could not tolerate the pain. By the end of June, Delores remained in pain and her family started making more frequent trips to her home to cover meals and help her around the house. Clara and Margo (a wonderful friend from our church) also pitched in some hours to help Delores, as they knew her needs well, were willing to help out, and she was open to their assistance. She kept thinking she would get better, but progress was slow, and despite all kinds of workups, there was no adequate explanation for why she was in such terrible pain and not healing better. She was having problems walking, and as her advocate, I felt like I was hitting a dead end. Every doctor told her she should be patient and that healing takes time. While she is typically optimistic, she began to feel like her independence was decreasing as her pain was increasing. Her appetite was not her normal level, and she felt frustrated. Eventually, she was put on low-level pain medications to help control the pain but not make her too unsteady when she did get up to walk. Falls are always a concern with these medications, along with her unsteadiness from the pain, a potentially lethal combination for any senior.

On July 6th, in the evening, her son called to tell me that Delores could not walk or bear weight on her left foot and her pain was unbearable. This was an acute change, as she had always been able to weight bear up until this time. I went over to evaluate her and decided with this sudden change, she needed to be evaluated at the hospital. I dialed 911 and the ambulance came. I had been overseeing her medical care for years, so I got in the ambulance with her. I knew Delores's medical history by heart and could give them the lowdown on what exactly had transpired with her over the previous two months and beyond.

In Montgomery County, Maryland, you can typically request to go to a certain hospital if the situation at hand is not a life-threatening emergency. I asked the young ambulance driver to take Delores to a community hospital five miles away, where all her doctors were, instead of the hospital one mile away. From a logistical standpoint, it made sense to send her where all her records were, along with her previous orthopedic surgeon. My request was denied, as the driver said to me, "She will get a pain pill and be home in two hours; you watch." While I did not agree with the driver, I opted to not argue with him, and against my wishes, we went to the local hospital. At eighty-six and in severe pain, Delores did not appear anything like her baseline person who up until seven weeks ago only needed help with her transportation but maintained her own home alone, with the exception of errands and bill paying.

The doctor examined her, and his initial impression was that she had a kidney stone. He wanted a CT scan of the abdomen; I requested an X-ray of the hip and was told that the CT would show the left hip joint so we would cover both areas with one test. I accepted his explanation, as he was the doctor and this was his assessment. But I was confused because I had never seen a kidney stone present in this way. Delores was sent to radiology after being given copious amounts of pain medications, and we waited for the results. About two hours later, the CT scan report was ready and the doctor came back telling us that there was no kidney stone. I asked about the hip, and he said, "Initially, it looked like there was an issue in her joint, but it was reviewed again and it is fine."

When he told me that they would like to put Delores on the twenty-three-hour observation unit for pain management, I spoke up and told him whatever was troubling her, twenty-three hours would not be enough time to address it. He did listen to me and Delores was admitted to a unit in the hospital for pain management and observation for a yet undetermined cause. As is typically the case, we brought in a caregiver to be at the bedside for Delores should she need help during the night. But the mystery remained, what was wrong with Delores?

We contacted a very good orthopedic surgeon whom we knew and trusted, and I told him the details of Delores's situation. The next morning I was paged overhead to the radiology department after the doctor read the X-ray of her left hip. The orthopedic surgeon met me there and told me the head of Delores's left femur had snapped off and was no longer attached to the bone; thus, she would need hip replacement surgery as soon as possible. His theory was that the head of the femur must have broken off around the time that Delores could no longer bear weight. There was no fall, but there was a significant fracture possibly due to her being on steroids for Addison's disease since 2008. Long-term use of steroids can contribute to AVN, which is the death of bone tissue due to lack of blood flow, and the cause of her first hip replacement in 2008. At least we now had an answer and a plan.

As Delores was being prepared for surgery, I was told that some of her lab values were abnormal, and they would need to be corrected prior to having surgery. I was not made aware of this in the emergency room and did not know until learning the surgery would be delayed. It took forty-eight hours to get her labs corrected, and on Tuesday night (the 9th), she was scheduled for surgery, but it had to be canceled again, this time due to low blood pressure. The next day, Delores went into surgery for her hip replacement. Her family and concerned friends took over the waiting room, and two hours later when the doctor came out with good news, we were all very relieved. It seemed Delores was on her way to recovery. The words "She will be home in two hours after a pain pill . . ." kept replaying in my mind. We were beyond frustrated. Since May 12th Delores had been in increasing pain with no explanation; it was clear these two months had taken a toll on her body physically, as she was struggling with new medical issues. To say it had been a long two months would be an understatement.

So, we were extra relieved to get the good news, but sometimes the stars just don't seem to align and this was definitely one of those times. An hour after surgery, when she was in the recovery room, Delores's vital signs began to change and her pulse began to climb higher. The rapid response team came and diagnosed her with atrial fibrillation. She was admitted to the IMCU for cardiac monitoring because of her new cardiac issues. However, this was not optimal because they were not accustomed to having fresh orthopedic post-op patients on their unit and were unfamiliar with the management of a hip replacement patient. Atrial fibrillation (A-fib) can happen at any time, so there was no direct known cause for this occurring, but the prior two months of extreme pain, debility, and stress may have played a role in Delores developing this condition. Once atrial fibrillation is diagnosed, the risk becomes high for a stroke or heart attack due to the potential of blood clots. In new cases of A-fib, the physicians like to try and convert the heart back into a normal rhythm if they can (cardiac ablation). Her heart rate was now very high (120–160 beats/min) and contributing to her ongoing exhaustion and shortness of breath. She felt as if she were running a marathon each and every hour. She could hardly hold her head up to speak, and she was pale, weak, and listless. I tried hard to remain optimistic, but the cards seemed to be stacked against her, and we knew that her prognosis was uncertain. The new onset of complications definitely prolongs recovery for patients.

I began to have multiple concerns with the quality of care that Delores was receiving in the hospital. For one, we had problems with infection control protocols; the floor in the room was filthy and stained with dirt and blood from the patient before. We even had a nurse use her same gloves for bathing Delores, changing her IV, and then putting a pill in her mouth. Delores, a nurse since the 1950s, actually called the nurse out when she did this, but the nurse became very defensive. She told the nurse, "You just put a pill in my mouth with the same gloves you cleaned my bottom with?" There were four of us in the room so what took place was clear and Delores was right. Another time, a nurse and I were repositioning Delores in the bed, and when she saw the bandage on Delores's thigh, she asked me, "Why is that bandage there?" I asked the nurse to step into the hall so I could explain that Delores had had a hip replacement, which was why she was in the hospital, but subsequently had developed A-fib which brought her to the cardiac step-down unit. The nurse explained she was late for her shift and never got the report, so she did not know what Delores was in the hospital for. I was so surprised, but again this goes back to this unit being a specialized cardiac unit, not an orthopedic unit. We even had a nurse who, while giving Delores care, kept pointing to her own mouth, and when I asked her what was wrong, she told me, "I need to go feed my face. I'm hungry," and proceeded to walk out have lunch and return thirty minutes later to finish changing Delores. Needless to say, the frustration continued.

I found it difficult to advocate for Delores's best interest while not being adversarial with the professional staff around me, who were truly trying to do their best. Hospital environments are high stress for medical providers, nurses, and techs; there is so much to do and only so much time to do it, and meeting every patient's needs is difficult when you are stretched so thin. I even enlisted the help of a dear friend Nurse Terry, who worked in the hospital, to consult with me and make sure that I was not being unreasonable with my expectations. Though she did not feel I was, she was called out by the staff of the hospital for getting "too involved" in our situation with Delores. It was to date my toughest advocacy case yet. I felt like each time I would try to address one issue, another issue came up. I felt like I was not being efficient in any way for Delores. I was stressed out, trying to work my regular job, trying to navigate difficult waters as an advocate, and being met with constant roadblocks and poor care. It took two months to get an answer, I could not redirect the ambulance to the hospital of Delores's choice, she was assumed to have a kidney stone when her femur was actually broken, and now she was in a cardiac unit where the staff was having a hard time managing her situation.

Delores began having more and more medical complications. She again developed a problem with her sodium level dropping and, in turn, her blood pressure dropped. The hospital doctors didn't order a dietary consult or create a treatment plan to rectify this drop. Her albumin level dropped to a dangerous level. Without proper albumin, the building blocks of protein levels, patients cannot heal.

On July 17th, I was told that Delores had been diagnosed with a blood clot on the 14th. It was in her chart but not communicated to us until three days later. Her right arm had gotten very tender and sore. She then developed diarrhea, she was weakening, and her medication list was growing with more and more serious medications with an increased potential for side effects and drug–drug interactions. On the 17th, Delores was taken for her cardiac ablation (second surgery), and fortunately, her heart went back to a regular rhythm for her after twelve days of beating at 120–160 beats per minute. One of the causes of her extreme exhaustion was now removed, and our hope was that her heart would stay in a normal rhythm at her normal 70–80 beats per minute. But the odds were mounting, and her situation was much more complex than when she was admitted.

On the 19th, we were told that Delores had an infection in her left hip incision and antibiotics were added to the mix. I requested that Delores get moved to the orthopedic unit, as she had not been out of bed for twelve days now, but the nurses were concerned about moving her as they were not trained for orthopedic patients. Luckily, the cardiologist approved the move. Within five minutes, there was a knock at Delores's door and a transport person with a wheelchair was standing there. We were happy with how quickly this request was made only to find out that the hospitalist misunderstood my request and thought that I had asked that Delores be taken to the garden outside. Communication was a problem.

Around 11 p.m., one of Delores's sons came, and she was moved to the orthopedic unit, which was good as now we could have them focus on getting her up and moving. The next day, we were told that Delores would need to have another surgery to open up the surgical wound and clean it out, a process known as "debridement." Her third surgery was done on a Sunday, as the physician did not feel it should wait, so he took time out of his busy weekend to attend to Delores and her now-aggressive infection. He was aware of our frustrations and was deeply empathetic to her situation. He was also frustrated, as he had wanted her out of bed long before then. Her immobility contributed to her post-op complications, not to mention the lack of experience the cardiac unit of the hospital had in dealing with post-op orthopedic patients.

On the 24th, we were told that another surgery would be needed to open up the incision again, and this time they would need to remove the prosthetic hip. By this time Delores was not doing well, and I felt like she was beginning to "circle the drain." There was not much optimism from any of her medical providers that her outcome would be good, due to all of her mounting complications. We understood that it may be her "time" but were so frustrated by all the complications and miscommunications that had compounded her issues.

As Delores faced her fourth surgery, Delores's youngest son, Curt, called his close friend from high school and told him about his mother's situation and how dire it was looking. While I was seeing patients in the GI office adjacent to the hospital, I got a call from this family friend in Wyoming who was also an orthopedic surgeon. He suggested that given all the complications and stressors Delores was facing, we move her to another hospital to see an orthopedic specialist who specialized in complicated infections in prosthetics (hip and knee joints). I only knew one such doctor, who I had met with my advocacy client Jeffrey a few years prior, and he was located in Virginia. I was able to call him, get right through to him, and explain the entire situation. He said he would be happy to handle the case as he dealt with MRSA infections all the time and felt very comfortable with his hospital in Virginia. It was one of the hardest things I have ever had to do, but we were able to move Delores to Virginia by ambulance at 8 p.m. that night. The local orthopedic surgeon understood our plight, as he too had been very disappointed by the care Delores received, and did not discourage the transfer. I told my full-time job that I would need to take a leave of absence to manage the situation with Delores. At this point I felt fairly certain that we would lose her, but moving her was a last-ditch effort and I had to be available for her in this time of need, not knowing if she would live or die. It was no one's fault that we were at this juncture, but my medical insight said to go for it.

That evening, she was rolled in through the ER, admitted, and sent up to her room. Because of her infection, she was in a private room that the case manager from the hospital had set up, and all the particulars were perfectly executed. By 11 p.m. she had been given a bag lunch to eat because she would not be able to have breakfast, labs were done, EKG was done, a catheter was inserted, and Delores went to sleep. Again, she was never left alone in the hospital, especially this hospital over an hour from home. Twenty days and three surgeries later, I thought of those ill-conceived words: "She will get a pain pill and be home in two hours."

On the 27th, this specialized orthopedic surgeon, Dr. G. and his team operated on Delores. He told us that he felt he could successfully treat the infection, and he would be monitoring the situation very carefully.

Delores was in good hands and this experience started off on the right foot. I was beginning to feel that she may pull out of this after all. However, she was not out of the woods yet. On the 29th, Delores was complaining of a new pain with any movement of her left leg. An X-ray was quickly ordered and it revealed a dislocation of the prosthesis. On the morning of the 30th, Delores called me to tell me that she was heading to surgery and, for the first time, expressed true fear. I called her chaplain to comfort her at her bedside, and he said a prayer with her. I was on my way to work when I decided to make a U-turn and go to Virginia to be with Delores. Juggling my full-time work as a nurse practitioner and my part-time advocacy job was definitely stressful, but the fifty-minute drive helped me to clear my head and determine what my focus was for the day as it related to Delores and her needs.

She got through her fifth surgery with no issues but was told she could not bear weight on that leg until further notice. The next morning, she was very anemic and received two units of packed red blood cells. She was exhausted, had not eaten all day, and she started having some confusion, asking me, "When will I be back on Earth?" Keeping caregivers with her each evening was so helpful so they could calm her, as she had been through so much and reassurance is truly not a task the hospital's nursing staff had the time to provide. The investment was worth her reassurance and our peace of mind. This confusion is called Delirium and is prompted by the acute illness affecting patients in the hospital and increases the risk of falling as they sometimes try to get out of bed in their weakened conditions.

By the first of August, she was feeling a bit better after the blood transfusions and improved sleep. She told me, "I think I am going to make it." This was great to hear. But these words revealed to me for the first time that she had possibly been thinking about not recovering. It had been almost four weeks since she went to the ER, but actually three months since her fall. Around this time, it was determined that she not only had an MRSA infection but that she was now also growing fungus in her bloodstream as well. A very strong anti-fungal medication was started.

She was up and down over the course of the next four days.

She went on to have two more surgeries, for a total of seven.

She also developed "red man syndrome," which is a terrible rash that turns the patient's whole body red, is itchy, and makes them feel absolutely miserable, as if their skin is hot and on fire.

On the 12th, Delores was released to bear weight on her left leg, and she called and left a very excited voicemail that she "walked eighteen steps today." The rash was starting to dissipate, but she was on heavy doses of steroids. Her emotions went from confusion to elation and fear/fright to joy. The roller coaster ride continued.

On the 15th, Delores was transferred to the cardiac unit on the sixth floor, due to her cardiac issues that required closer monitoring. On the 16th, as I drove to Virginia, I thought about the events of Delores's medical issues since May and decided that perhaps we should discuss hospice care. As I drove from work in Maryland to Virginia, I rehearsed the difficult words I would say to her when I saw her. When I entered the room, she said she needed to talk to me. I told her that I also wanted to talk to her but that she should go first. Delores said, "I am ready to get out of here. I have my granddaughter Dara's wedding to get to. I need to start walking, and I need a dress." This was music to my ears. I opted to put the hospice discussion on the back burner; why take away her optimism at this point? This was the confirmation we needed to hear from Delores after a grueling six-week journey. Her will was engaged and she was feeling very positive, as were we, about her recovery.

On September 2nd, 2014, Delores came home, after an amazing journey, with a renewed appreciation for life. She also now required full-time 24/7 help in her home, as she was still in physical therapy, had a wound vacuum, and she needed help navigating around wherever she went with the walker. Her will had won and she was on her way to continuing to enjoy the life she loved. Though she now needed more care, she was home and that was what mattered most. We brought in fantastic caregivers to help Delores.

Home health care provided amazing help in the home with all her medical needs. Delores's "village" was a huge part of her recovery. So many family and friends came to Virginia and encouraged her along the way, giving her hope and leaving her with words of inspiration. Once she was home, meals were delivered, treats were dropped off, and friends continued to stream in and lift her spirits. Family filled her home with laughter again, and about a year later, Delores was almost back to her baseline. Delores knew she had dodged a myriad of bullets and was grateful for every single day. As her advocate, I was grateful for the lines of communication remaining open and for the advice of the friend in Wyoming who had encouraged me to step out of my comfort zone and transfer Delores at a very difficult time.

Breaking down each issue one at a time was helpful for clarity. As her advocate, I knew this would be a tough road but never anticipated just how arduous it could be. Again, I learned to not give up hope even if it looks fateful. I learned to not always look at the big picture, but rather break it down to day by day and notice the small victories. I knew that this could be the end of Delores's story, but I wanted that to be of natural causation and not because there was a system failure. While it was very extreme to move Delores to another state, it was done as a last-ditch effort, and if she was going to succumb, we wanted to make sure we explored every option. I had a huge village behind me with the rest of Delores's family, who were tuned in every step of the way. Hope, prayer, and optimism were the wind in her sails that she relied on as much as the medical professionals in her life.

Outcome:

Delores got to attend her granddaughter Dara's wedding in a wheelchair that September, accompanied by her caregiver, Evelyn, and surrounded by her loving family. She held her eldest great-granddaughter, Finlee, who was just four months old, on her lap. She was feeling strong and able to endure the entire wedding, reception, and evening very well. She remained in her single-family home with 24/7 caregivers who helped strengthen her, assist her with activities of daily living, and provide safety while recovering. After four months, she was able to reduce these hours to two days a week for four hours a day, thanks to Margo and Clara. They paid her bills, kept her home clean, and made sure Delores could be comfortable in her home. Her stair climber allowed her to stay up in her bedroom despite her son Jeff working tirelessly to put in a full bath next to the bedroom on the main floor. She wanted to sleep upstairs, and she did! She had a strong will and remained very much in control but did defer to me for any health concerns that arose.

She again got back into her community programs like garden club and support groups, but her eyesight continued to decline, and in December 2016, during a flight to Florida, she lost her hearing in her left ear. This was, of course, a blow as she had always said that although her vision was so poor, she was so grateful for her hearing. Her hearing was diminished to only 25 percent in her left ear. While this was a huge disappointment to her, she found the ability to overcome this new challenge and continue to "love life." Her attitude and passion for life continued to propel her forward through each day.

Advocacy tips:

- You need to remember to put your foot down. Had I put my foot down about sending her to the hospital with doctors who knew her, there most likely wouldn't have been a delay in her diagnosis.
- You need to always stay on top of every issue that arises, even if it is arduous to do so.
- Because it is important to keep in communication with the physicians, which can be hard to do with their erratic schedules, always keep someone at the bedside who can communicate with you.
- Sometimes you have to take big leaps of faith. Moving from our local hospital to Virginia was a leap of faith but one that I am so glad we did.

· Chapter 10 ·

Grandpop-Us Versus Them

"Patience is the calm acceptance that things can happen in a different order than the one you have in mind."

—David G. Allen

On a cold winter Saturday morning in January 2015, we got a call from our middle son who was at college in Pennsylvania. He explained that he had gotten a Facebook message from a total stranger from NYC asking if he was related to Richard Kohn. He responded "yes," that he was in fact his grandpop. The stranger, who turned out to be Richard's good friend, Mangus, gave him an ominous message: "He is in trouble." Our son, who was twenty at the time, called us immediately and relayed this concerning message to us.

We swung into action and, of course, tried to call Richard to no avail. We didn't waste any time and reached out to the police department in upper Manhattan. They told us they would do a wellness check and get back to us. About an hour later we got a call from the police, who told us that Richard was in his apartment, on the floor, alive but very weak and frail. They transported him to the hospital but weren't certain he would survive the ride to the hospital.

We then called our eldest son, Matthew, who lived in Brooklyn, and he was soon on his way to meet his grandfather at the emergency room. Our son had moved to Brooklyn the previous September for a job. He had been very diligent about being in touch with his grandfather, and they tried to meet for lunch about once a week. It was a wonderful time for Matthew and his grandfather as they got to connect on a different level while they were both living in New York City. However, since he knew his grandfather had not been feeling well and that he had a "cold," he had canceled their lunch the previous week. Matthew didn't think too much of his grandfather not answering his calls; his grandpop was an actor and often did short gigs all over the city, so he simply thought Grandpop was busy and would get back to him when he could.

Now Matthew was sitting with his grandpop at his bedside in a very cramped ER in the middle of New York

City. Grandpop had a bruise that extended down the entire right side of his face and all the way down his body from lying on the floor for what appeared to be many days, perhaps as many as five. There were so many unanswered questions, as Grandpop was eighty years old, lived on his own, and the last person to speak to him was the Facebook stranger who reached out to Matthew's brother at college. It was a scary time for Matthew to be in the ER alone with his grandfather, who clearly was in rough shape.

While he was alive, his kidneys were in shock due to the ramifications of a fall and lying on the floor for so long. He needed scans of his entire body to determine the damage from the fall. Grandpop had lived alone, was very independent, and loved his NYC lifestyle, so this was undoubtedly upsetting to him. Matt's presence was a godsend. Grandpop was unable to speak intelligibly, but knew Matt was with him. But speech didn't matter, as Matt was there to hold his hand. Human touch can sometimes replace words, as touch conveys love and caring when there simply are no words.

In the meantime, we quickly booked an Amtrak train from Rockville, Maryland, and went to the Big Apple with our youngest son in tow. It was an eerie train ride, unsure of what awaited us in New York with our beloved grandpop. But there was a level of comfort in knowing that Matthew was at the bedside and Grandpop was not alone. The timing of Matthew's first job, his renewed relationship with his grandfather, and the ability to get to him so quickly were reassuring to us.

We arrived at the hospital about five hours later. The doctors admitted him to the hospital, and we would be there to support him through this difficult time. The doctors could not explain how or why Grandpop had fallen, but both a heart attack and stroke had been ruled out as the culprit. We were told that the scans and tests were all clear. His blood work was very abnormal, and he needed intravenous fluids and medications to slowly rehydrate him and try to get his labs back to a normal baseline.

Before we left the hospital that night, it was clear that if Grandpop needed resuscitation for any reason, he would not have the invasive and traumatic chest compressions per his written advanced directives; this is called Do Not Resuscitate (DNR). His condition was so weak from the previous five days that we knew he could not survive this, and it would add to his discomfort. We left the hospital in the middle of the night and went back to his apartment.

The first night in NYC we were awakened by a phone call from the doctor at the hospital telling us that Grandpop had a stroke during the night that caused a pretty large area of hemorrhage on the left side of the brain, but we were hopeful that with immediate treatment, he would improve with minimal residual impact. Unfortunately, due to his weakened fragile condition, he was unable to obtain the "clot-busting" medication that is sometimes given to reverse the damage of a stroke.

The next day we saw Grandpop in the ICU. Though he was still unable to speak, he did try. He was unable to swallow, and he could not move his right arm or leg, a change from when he first arrived at the ER. He also could not open his right eye. Despite the stroke, he was relatively stable until he began to bleed internally from his GI tract, most likely his stomach. We had a family meeting with the palliative care team about his status. He was debilitated from the fall that left him in the same position for days, compromised from a stroke, and now suffered a GI bleed. His prognosis was not good. We reviewed his advanced directives and reached out to his ex-wife for confirmation of his decision. She reminded us that his mother had a stroke similar to this and was in a nursing home for five years, tube-fed and turned every two hours, and this was a fate that Richard wanted to avoid: he had clearly stated that "he never wanted to live like his mother did her last five years." Steve, Richard's only surviving kin, was given all the facts of the situation, and it was his decision to honor his father's wishes. That evening, we were visited by a physician who explained to us that in his current condition, if Richard were intubated for any reason, he likely would not be extubated after the procedure due to his fragile nature. He gave us good insight and was honest with us.

While I had a pretty good understanding of Richard's frail condition, I wanted my husband to be fully informed of the whole situation and then make the final decision based upon his father's wishes and the medical facts. Compounding the situation, Grandpop's albumin level was low, his nutritional status was poor, he had many wounds on his body, and he was bleeding internally. I explained to Steve what I understood was going on with his father, reviewed all the labs, and had many discussions with the ICU physicians to clarify any questions that we had. We had a palliative care meeting, and it was quite clear that the room was split down the middle regarding Steve's decision to honor Richard's advanced directives. The intensivists were in favor of doing everything in their power to keep Richard alive at any cost. In fact, after the meeting, some physicians came into the room and made some comments that clearly were in deference to what Steve had decided based on his father's desires. There was definitely a feeling that it was "us vs. them": the physicians who wanted to save Richard vs. the physicians who saw that Richard's health issues were complex and difficult to recover from. This felt very conflictual to us, so we had the palliative physician paged to come speak to us to clarify our feelings of conflict. The physician returned to the ICU and told us that this decision was the right decision for someone in this debilitating condition, and if, in fact, Richard did survive, he would need care 24/7, need to be turned every two hours, and tube-fed for the rest of his life.

The intensivists were not thrilled with Steve's final decision, and when asked about intubation, Steve was clear that he wanted his father to remain a DNI (do not intubate). Despite the DNI directive, the respiratory therapist came in to set up a ventilator. When Steve asked why he was setting up the ventilator, he told us that Richard was supposed to have a procedure known as an EGD, where they were going to look down his esophagus and stomach to see where the GI bleed was coming from, and this procedure required him to be intubated. Steve repeated that his father was not to be intubated. Again, this was a very uneasy feeling, as he felt judged for a decision that he painstakingly made with education and advice from experts.

They finally honored Richard's advanced directives, and on day four said that if this was the final decision, that hospice was appropriate for Richard. A hospice consult was done and a nurse from Bellevue Hospital came to talk to us and see Richard. A transfer was put in for the following morning.

On a cold winter morning, we covered Grandpop, who wore his hospital gown, with warm blankets and a wool stocking cap, and Steve, Matthew, and I jammed into the ambulette with Richard and all our suitcases for the long journey down to the Lower East Side. It felt surreal to drive through New York City, knowing it was Grandpop's last trip. This city had been his home for twenty years, ever since he started his second career as an actor at age sixty after a divorce. We were grateful he got to live out his dream, which his parents were never in favor of but that fueled a lifelong passion. In retrospect, so many positives came from Richard's life, but the part that resonated with me was that he and his twenty-two-year-old grandson formed a bond in the last eighteen months of his life that they would not have been able to do if Matt had not gotten a job in New York City. In Richard's eulogy, Matthew talked about how he never had a desire to go to NYC, but he was intrigued by a job offer that took him there. He met his Grandpop for lunch routinely and kibitzed about life, adventures, and acting as a second career. Grandpop developed a very close personal relationship with his eldest grandson. Matthew felt that this opportunity in New York was not just the start of his career but a gift of added time to be in the same city with his grandfather and enjoy these last eighteen months with him.

Grandpop was in hospice in Bellevue Hospital, in a unit designated for only end-of-life patients. They did a great job of making the unit very comfortable. They made it more like a hotel than a hospital stay: pets came to visit the patients and musicians would come and play music for them. For five days the family stayed with Grandpop, day and night, at hospice, then he took his last breath on February 3rd, 2015, with his family by his side. He was at peace and his end-of-life wish was fulfilled.

Outcome:

We were able to meet the stranger who reached out to Chris over Facebook. He was a fellow actor who did many gigs with Grandpop. He was about twenty years his junior but was a very good friend to him. He told us that he had spoken with Richard on Monday and noted that he did not sound good. He had encouraged him to go see his doctor, but he could not reach him again to see if he actually went. On Saturday, he had a sinking feeling, and that is when he reached out on Facebook to try and find a relative of Grandpop's. We told him how much we appreciated the friendship he shared with Grandpop and how grateful we were that we had the gift of ten more days with him where we could tell him how much we loved him and keep him company as he transitioned from this Earth. If Mangus had not contacted our son on Facebook, Grandpop would have most likely died alone in his apartment. We felt such gratitude that we could be with him.

Advocacy tips:

- Make sure you hold your ground when it comes to honoring the dying wishes of a loved one. Don't worry about being "judged" by any of the doctors or nurses; they don't have to agree with your decision. While people can "survive" such catastrophic injuries, the question becomes what type of quality of life do they end up with? This is why writing down your advanced directives ahead of time is so pivotal in being proactive in a situation like this.

- Stay informed so you can present your case from an informed medical standpoint. Having all the lab results in front of us and knowing all the hurdles he would need to overcome before he got to an "acceptable" level for discharge was helpful. One doctor said to us "most families are not as informed of all the complexities of this situation as you are." We knew Grandpop wanted to be DNR, and the DNI was something we were able to deduce from Leah.

- Always hold your ground when it comes to making the best decision for a loved one.

· Chapter 11 ·

Finally an Answer

"Don't set your mind on things you don't possess as if they were yours, but count the blessings you actually possess and think how much you would desire them if they weren't already yours."

—Marcus Aurelius

Anna had been struggling for more than a year. At nineteen, she suffered from stomach bloating, nausea, abdominal pain, diarrhea, and vomiting after eating. Her menstrual cycle was painful and very irregular. Her skin was breaking out and caused her to spend a considerable amount of money on creams, washes, and treatments that did nothing to help her. In addition, her hair became thin and seemed to almost stop growing. All this equated to a rather significant weight loss, a depressed mood, lack of motivation, and incapacitating headaches. She started seeing her primary care provider (PCP) and was initially told she had a summer flu, so she should eat toast and applesauce. It didn't help.

Before she got sick, she had just left home to live on her own while attending a local community college. Within a week of telling her she should eat toast, her PCP diagnosed her with a "stress reaction" and gave her a prescription for Xanax. Her stomach felt as if it were on fire, almost like being dipped in acid from all the vomiting, reflux, and inflammation. Given her symptoms, they ordered a stool sample, which was then subsequently lost. As things progressed, she ended up in the ER where the workup was cursory and no definitive diagnosis was given. She was told to again follow up with her PCP. She did as she was told, and she felt as if her PCP and staff thought she had a case of hypochondriasis (a condition in which an individual is excessively and unduly worried about having a serious illness), mixed with depression and possibly an eating disorder.

In desperation, her mother reached out to me, and I facilitated an appointment to have her evaluated and subsequently scoped with blood work done in the GI office where I was working at the time. The scope procedure of her esophagus, stomach, and part of her small intestine, called an esophagogastroduodenoscopy (EGD), showed evidence of celiac disease (an autoimmune process that affects the small intestine whereby gluten is difficult to digest and can cause a myriad of symptoms), a surplus of inflammation, and a medical explanation for her supposed hypochondriasis. The EGD showed actual blunting of the cilia in the lining of the stomach.

The results of the EGD prompted her to go on a limited diet. After implementing a diet free of dairy, gluten, soy, and eggs, this young woman moved forward with her life.

Xanax did not prove to be the answer but could have perpetuated an addiction that is hard to break. Xanax belongs to a class of medications called Benzodiazepines; they are highly addictive and very similar to alcohol in the way they make you feel. This situation with Anna could have become much more complicated by adding psychotropic medications that she not only did not need but did nothing to address her issues. We are so quick to put teenagers on a medication that simply "Band-Aids" the problem and makes them "mentally less affected by it" so they don't perceive there to be as much of a problem. This can potentially lead to many additional issues, not to mention "polypharmacy," which is the concurrent use of multiple medications by a patient, which may or may not even address the initial problem. The use of polypharmacy, in fact, increases the risk of medication interactions and can cause interactions or even mask much bigger issues.

Food sensitivities are very common but are complete game changers for people who have them. In our GI practice, it was amazing how many people would come to find out that they simply did not break down certain foods "normally," and finding this out helped change lives forever, like in Anna's case.

Outcome:

Fast forward ten years, Anna is now a healthy, active, married mother of two who is thriving in life as long as she sticks to her dietary restrictions. All symptoms have abated with the exception of some bloating, stomach pains, and diarrhea if she happens to eat something outside of her restrictions. This is not always a willful occurrence, as an occasional meal outside the home can cause these symptoms when she is not completely aware of ingredients. It is hard to be invited out to friends' homes and question each food item and what is in it, but if she doesn't, she will pay for it and will know immediately that something she ate contained one of the ingredients that her system does not tolerate.

Advocacy tips :

- PCPs are very good gatekeepers, but when appropriate, you should reach out to specialists, or you might find they start treating the patient for depression or other mental illnesses that not only can perpetuate an addiction but do NOT fix the problem that they came into the office for in the first place.
- Do not give up if you don't get answers from your PCP. Many insurance companies will allow you to see a specialist to address additional health concerns.

- Trust your gut and listen to your patient, family, or loved one. It is amazing how much of the story and severity of a situation can be assessed by active listening. Get the story, write down the facts, tease out variables, and then decide if further action needs to be taken. Do not hesitate to reach out to a medical professional for advice or even other people who have had the same problem as they can often lead you to a solution.
- Ask questions. Ask about the efficacy of medications and about options. Benzodiazepines happen to be misused frequently in our society and should be prescribed judiciously. While mental health issues can cause physiological problems, be careful not to determine a psychological cause of a symptom without a proper workup.

· Chapter 12 ·

His and Hers

*"Life is ten percent what you experience and ninety percent how
you respond to it."*

—Dorothy M. Neddermeyer

Flo and I have been dear friends since 1995, busy raising our children but continuing to share life experiences
and tips for raising healthy families. Flo, a college athlete,
met her husband, Mo, on the volleyball court. They raised
three active children similar in age to our three sons. But
they were much more athletically focused, as Mo was the

women's volleyball coach for a local university in town. This couple has used volleyball to help shape young ladies into women of character and strength. Through this sport, they had worldwide opportunities. Mo has always stated, "I play games for a living." He has been very successful and won many awards with international recognition for his accomplishments as a coach, and his wife, Flo, has been by his side every step of the way. She has been able to accompany him on trips all over the world to recruit talented players, meet with families, and support his college team for over thirty years. In the midst of his career, they also raised three talented children who each excelled at the collegiate level with their own athletic abilities.

Flo had a difficult childhood related to asthma and frequent illnesses that kept her out of school until she was eight years old. I was unaware of Flo's unhealthy childhood, as she seemed like the picture of health to me other than the typical colds, viruses, and sore throats. She had no surgeries as a child. But Flo recalls "rapid heartbeats" as far back as her college days, and even as she raised her children, she would have "episodes" when she would tell the children that she needed a glass of water, assuming dehydration was the cause, and then would lie down until the episode passed. She had routine checkups her whole life. Once her husband took a job, her medical care was overseen by a managed care group. Though she would report these episodes of rapid heartbeats, no professionals, including several cardiologists, could give her a good explanation. She left the managed care group after her daughter had surgery that Flo felt was mismanaged, and switched their insurance to a large traditional insurance company PPO, which in hindsight afforded her some excellent new options and oversight of her health.

In 2010, Flo had an "episode," but it was a bit different from her rapid heartbeats in the past. This incident occurred at a fancy restaurant in the city where they were celebrating a large sports event. This time around she had sudden nausea, vomiting, and syncope (fainting) that landed her in the emergency room where another workup did not reveal the reason for this sudden illness. She chalked it up to a very stressful several weeks related to this large event and went on about her business.

In early 2012, after another successful tournament weekend, she called me. This was the first time I became aware of her episodes, and she informed me that the day prior, she had had a sustained heart rate of 170 beats per minute for an eight-hour period until it finally slowed down to her normal pace. This episode was atypical for her as her usual remedy of lying down after drinking a glass of water did not alleviate the situation. I was quite alarmed by her symptoms. Although I have never worked in cardiology, I had the basic knowledge to know that a sustained heart rate at that level was a medical emergency. I told her that I felt that she should have been seen urgently to be monitored. She was rather dismissive but did hear my alarmed tone. She told me that she was going to contact her husband's cardiology group as soon as she could get an appointment. But because she couldn't get an appointment for weeks with her husband's cardiologist, she agreed to have me set up an appointment with my cardiologist, and within twenty-four hours, she was seen.

She called me as soon as she got out of the appointment and was a bit flabbergasted by the news she had just been given. She told me the cardiologist found two holes in her heart! This is a condition known as atrial septal defect (ASD), a congenital defect in the wall of the atrium, and if the hole is very small, no surgical intervention is needed, but if the hole is large enough, surgery is required. The symptoms are minimal as a child, but by age thirty, adults may notice symptoms, such as shortness of breath; heart palpitations; rapid heartbeats; fatigue; swelling in the legs, feet, or abdomen; and heart murmurs. Considering she was forty-nine at the time, the cardiologist ordered a cardiac ablation in March and beta-blocker medication to help slow down the heart rate. The ablation did not suffice, and she was then scheduled for open heart surgery in Baltimore by a world-renowned cardiac surgeon.

Her atrium had one hole the size of a dime; the other one was much smaller. Since 30 percent of her blood flow went in the wrong direction, she experienced symptoms periodically (her "episodes"). The doctor told her that her heart was enlarged on one side, a condition known as cardiomyopathy. If left untreated, this would have led to a heart transplant or sudden death. Flo was scheduled for surgery and was operated on at Johns Hopkins University Hospital in May. The procedure was successful, and she was an inpatient for a week after the surgery. During this procedure, they needed to thread a catheter into her right groin for access to the heart vessels and did mention that she had a residual hematoma at the site but did not expect that to lead to any future problems. She recalled a funny delusion she had during this hospitalization as she was getting out of bed the first day post-op to sit in a chair, under the influence of pain medication. Even years later, she could describe in vivid detail both the sound and the vision of a large parade of Clydesdale horses coming toward her. Her family still teases her about this, and she can still hear and see those big, beautiful horses "parading" the halls of the hospital in her mind's eye. She was very grateful for the precision of the surgeon and a cardiologist who looked deeper to find an explanation, and in November 2012, she was given the green light to resume her normal busy life.

Life slowly went back to normal for Flo, and she was soon traveling the world again with her husband. On a beautiful October day in 2015, now fifty-two-year-old Flo, who was at Johns Hopkins University watching her son play college lacrosse, texted me from the bathroom. She told me that she hadn't felt well all morning and was having terrible pain in what she described as the right lower quadrant of her abdomen. I was supposed to head up and watch the game myself. "Bring some drugs; I've got major cramping for some reason," she texted me. "I feel like I am in labor.

deeper into her symptoms and find a cause. During surgery, it was determined that the hematoma in her groin had adhered to her intestine and caused it to twist and cut off blood supply to a portion of her bowel, which was the reason for the severe pain. The area without blood flow was not viable and became necrotic (dead tissue). Thankfully, she only had to have several inches of her bowel removed. Her bowel was resected and no colostomy was needed. By the grace of God, she luckily did not follow her gut and go home and crawl into her bed, as that could have had devastating results for her.

After another unplanned week recuperating in the hospital, she came home and slowly got back to her life and again was very grateful for excellent medical care, including a skilled trauma surgeon, excellent health care providers, and nurses to help her recover. Flo always amazed me in how she was the picture of health, yet when she had a medical issue, it was never simple.

Life got back to its normal excitement, full of adventures for Flo and Mo. Their children finished college, got married, and began having children. After Flo's experience with the cardiologist, who saved her life by properly diagnosing her, she convinced her husband to switch to the same practice. Over the 2019 Christmas holidays, Mo was supposed to see the doctor and have "routine blood work." With the chaos of the holidays, the labs were delayed and the appointment was postponed until January. In January, when he got in to see the cardiologist for his routine follow-up, she asked him how he had been feeling. He told her he felt fine and was just as busy as ever. The doctor told Mo that his calcium level had "changed a little bit, and [she was] not comfortable with it." Two days later Mo was scheduled for a cardiac catheterization, and during the procedure, the vascular surgeon said to him, "Whoever sent you here just saved your life. Your left anterior descending artery (LAD) is almost completely occluded, and you need a stent right now!"

Twenty-eight hours later, Flo and Mo left the hospital with excellent news, again skirting danger and filled with gratitude. Getting regular workups and seeing meticulous providers who took the time to listen, investigate, and refer to specialists when needed paid off once again. This cardiologist intervened once again and was now responsible for lifesaving procedures for both Flo and Mo.

Outcome:

Both Flo and Mo are enjoying good health and have realized the benefits of good medical care. They continue to take good care of themselves and get regular checkups. They are grateful that they were able to change health care plans when they did and understand the value of being heard by their doctors.

Early intervention made the difference for both of these wonderful humans, and they are enjoying their growing family as a result of their excellent health.

Advocacy tips:

As an advocate, I recommended highly regarded medical providers and encouraged intervention when I felt that it was needed. I am always happy when people ask my opinion and then take my advice. This comes from building a trusting relationship.

Make sure you establish rapport with your patients, and they will take your advice.

· Chapter 13 ·

Guy and Anita

"We don't know where we're going, we don't know what's going to happen, but no one can take away from you what you put in your own mind."

—Dr. Edith Eger

Anita and Guy, friends of our family who lived in Germany at the same time as we did and who also ended up relocating to Maryland in the late 1960s, reached out to me when Guy developed colon cancer. I became his medical advocate. I attended all his oncology appointments and his chemotherapy and radiation sessions. He was a beloved physician who practiced in the field of endocrinology and had a long-time practice in Washington, DC.

When he showed up at his office one day, his staff did not like his coloring and said he appeared to be weak and somewhat confused. Reluctantly, he was taken to the ER and found to be anemic with a dangerously low red blood cell count. He was admitted to the hospital, and during the course of the hospitalization, they found he had stage-4 colon cancer, which was the cause of his anemia. Not one to give up easily, he took on the fighting spirit. His children asked me to be his medical advocate as they were busy working and raising families and did not have the time to be available to help him. The girls were very close to their father and were very concerned that he get the best care available. They knew that their mother would not be able to help him as she had a long history of chronic debilitating mental illness.

Guy was a wonderful man and accompanying him to his appointments became a weekly event that I looked forward to. If by chance I could not make the appointment, I had two nurses, who also knew Guy very well, who would step in to help me, along with his devoted team of caregivers. We became a cohesive unit, and his medical providers worked closely with us to care for Guy. At his weekly meetings, Guy's caregiver would also come and provide important feedback about how he was doing as it related to his appetite, his weight, elimination patterns, vital signs, pain levels, and any other update that was crucial each week. He had a caregiver who was attentive and first-class. Eventually, we added more caregivers as Guy's needs increased, and they all grew close to him and Anita. They would make certain that medications were taken and that Guy was well fed and hydrated. Guy was in need of constant medication adjustments, and the oncologist adjusted steroids almost weekly based on what was going on with him.

During my initial in-home assessment, I asked how Anita was doing. The daughters told me that she was not really "in the picture" because of her mental health issues. They said the reason I did not know Anita very well was that since they were small children, she was really not a "present mother." She was always in her room lying down and never felt well. They had to walk on eggshells as she did not like noise. Because of this, they gravitated to their father to get most of their physical, mental, and emotional needs met. He was a very busy physician, so his plate was quite full providing for his family and playing both parental roles to the girls as they were growing up. One day their oldest daughter, Mary, said, "Pretend she is not here. You won't get anywhere with her!"

I had a hard time with this and left an open-ended assessment on the "spouse" section for Guy. These two had been married over fifty years when Guy got sick. He was so kind and so complimentary of his bride. Never did he utter anything about Anita that was not positive, but the girls definitely presented a different viewpoint.

I longed to work with Anita and felt that Guy could use his wife's support. But remembering what the girls told me, I felt torn. One day, Anita was awake and in the kitchen. I sat down with her and got to talking about what was going on with Guy. She told me how scared she was; after all, what would she ever do if her husband, who she relied on for everything, was no longer here one day? She began to converse, and I allowed her to talk freely about how she was feeling. As I started asking her open-ended questions, we developed a trusting relationship that, while initially forbidden, became one of the most trusting and satisfying patient relationships I have had. She was open, transparent, and trusted me. She had self-medicated for years with alcohol and over-the-counter pills to "help her nerves." She typically only came out of her dark bedroom for two hours a day from 6-8 p.m.

When I discovered she had been in therapy for years and had been seeing the same psychiatrist weekly for over twenty-five years, I asked her if she would be open to seeing a different psychiatrist that I had referred many patients to, and she said she would. We were making baby steps. Now I was advocating for both Anita and Guy. I was hoping that by helping Anita, I could help Guy and his daughters. This became part of my goals for this family.

Sometimes difficult conversations need to happen between family members or patients and me. I always strive to make these discussions as beneficial as possible to everyone, ensuring there are never any regrets when the patient's life ends. Part of helping people make decisions is to help them find the right specialist or provider who "speaks their language" and communicates effectively to their individualized needs. Since medical providers display a wide variety of bedside manners, it is extremely important that the patient feels at ease with each provider and can develop a trust that will help when difficult decisions need to be made. If a patient does not feel comfortable and does not feel as though they can develop a trust with their provider, I often help them find one who does meet their needs and gives them the confidence required in order to work together.

Anita began seeing the new psychiatrist Dr. Q on a regular basis, and she became properly medicated and stopped drinking through an intensive local program, and within nine months, Anita was a different woman. She not only came out of her room but she also began to attend the appointments with Guy. She grew to become the spouse she had never been. She was supportive, engaging, and concerned about her spouse. While things were looking up, she had some rough spots along the way. One night Anita called me, screaming at 11p.m. I went to her and just sat with her, offering her reassurance. Another time she was ranting in the car on the way to see her husband, yelling that she wished she were dead. I reached out and put my arm on her back to reassure her, and she settled down. Sometimes therapeutic touch is all that someone needs during a rough moment. Her chronic lifelong depression was debilitating and pervasive in her family; she grew up with parents and a brother who all had chronic depression. Her sister died of suicide, and her mother became bedbound from her depression, which proved fatal for her. Her children grew up in the same environment as she did. This was a mitzvah for me and for them as she continued to emerge from and break the cycle of difficult mental illness.

Over the next two years, Guy had his ups and downs with treatments, but eventually, we all knew the end was coming, and one day, I was present when Guy looked at Anita and said to her, "Thank you for being the wife I needed when I needed it." It was so special to witness this bond grow and my secret goal for this family realized—even the daughters were astonished at the progress their mother had made, against all odds, over the previous two years. However, ironically, she got a bit too involved when she tried to manage his medications. I had to tell her that these were all being ordered by his oncologist, and she could not change them on her own. I marveled at the thought of how much she had changed during this time. Be careful what you wish for, I thought to myself.

Guy and Anita opted for him to stay home until his final day, and we were able to make the accommodations for this to happen. Hospice was on board and a great support to our caregiving team while we all cared for Guy as the end approached. The sons and grandchildren were all present with Guy and Anita as they bid farewell to their amazing father.

Outcome:

Anita, the woman who was fearful of her future as a widow, did very well after her husband passed. She got the proper treatment for her lifelong mental health issues, and now the woman who used to sleep all day and night often calls me at 8 a.m. bright-eyed and bushy-tailed to see how I am doing. She continues to see Dr. Q and is now married to a fellow physician who was a widow and used to work with Guy. More importantly, her personality has come to life to her children, grandchildren, and her stepchildren and their children. Seeing her reminds me to always be optimistic and to never give up. It has been a privilege for me and my company to work with this family. The caregivers still go to see her. She will be eighty next year and still has a tremendous amount of living to do.

When Guy died, he did so with dignity. He was ready, his family was ready, and he lived the best life he could right up until his final breath.

The oncologist and interventional radiologist who worked with Guy have been a steady source of referrals for our company. It was a pleasure to be on this advocacy team. It is heartwarming to see relationships develop, even in the midst of terminal cancer treatments, with the health care providers and their ancillary staff. Even the infusion nurses were amazing and extremely warm and hospitable not only to Guy but to his entire "care team." They always had a warm blanket, a cup of tea, or a snack if the patient felt shaky. Guy did so well, even with the long-term, high-level chemotherapy and immunotherapy. Fortunately, because the oncology team was always extremely proactive in anticipating potential side effects, Guy rarely ever experienced them and remained as comfortable as possible throughout his entire treatment regimen.

Advocacy tips:

- When your patient is in need of constant medication adjustments, these frequent changes can be time-consuming and need to be overseen by an experienced, licensed practitioner for legal reasons and to avoid potential mistakes. Also with these frequent changes, it is important that an RN, or licensed medical provider, accompany your patient to each visit and make the appropriate adjustments and ensure all notes are updated. This isn't a job for private caregivers. Ever-changing medications require careful monitoring and constant feedback to the doctors with frequent email correspondence.
- Communication with the family is pivotal to help them feel like a part of the care team for their loved one during their illness. With Guy, we kept a communication log book in the home for all caregivers and specialists, such as physical therapists, occupational therapists, and RNs, who came into the home and provided services for Guy.

- The privilege of working with a couple and their family is multifaceted and can be complicated. Each relationship and each family presents a multitude of obstacles and challenges. Thus, a customized family care plan is essential in assisting the care team to provide the most comprehensive care not only to the patient but to their entire family.

· Chapter 14 ·

The Baker Sisters and Adult Protective Services (APS)

"The greatest weapon against stress is our ability to choose one thought over another."

—William James

I got a call one afternoon from a social worker asking me if our company would take care of two sisters, Elsie and Mary Jo, who were in her long-term care facility but really wanted to go back home to live where they had shared a home together for over forty years. APS was involved and wanted to make sure that they had advocates and were properly cared for. I set up an assessment, met up with them, and did a tour of their home to determine if this was a feasible plan.

The home needed some work and a thorough cleaning to make it habitable. They needed help with getting their financial affairs in order, and they needed bills paid to restore electricity, cable, and all home necessities. And as it turned out, their mail had not been opened for two years; thus, checks were never cashed (including thousands of dollars of social security benefits checks) and all health and life insurance policies had been canceled.

Prior to their time in the long-term-care facility, these gals had been living alone. Elsie and Mary Jo had a brother who died of cancer about twenty years before we met them, and the sisters cared for him. Their mother and father aged in the home where they currently live and both sisters came home to nurse their parents until they died. They were both retired from government jobs and never married. Once their brother and both parents had passed away, it was just the two of them who suddenly found themselves aged and unable to care for their own needs but unaware of their situation. They were not opening their mail and managing a household was no longer possible, basically the "wheels started falling off the bus" so to speak. One sister was showing signs of cognitive decline; the other was showing signs of pretty deep depression, and she was the one who was "managing" all the finances. With no next of kin or friends who checked on the pair regularly, they were basically scraping by until one day when Elsie called 911 because Mary Jo couldn't move. The EMTs showed up, took a look around at the deplorable conditions, and decided very astutely that both Elsie and Mary Jo needed to be taken to the hospital. The hospital worked up Mary Jo for an acute infection and also cared for Elsie due to her diagnosis of "complicated social history." The sisters were then placed in a rehabilitation facility where APS began overseeing their complicated social history.

Now they wanted to go home. We began working with the sisters and got their home cleaned up and in good working order. We placed a caregiver in their home to oversee their care, medications, and all aspects of their life. The true hero in this story is a woman named Jeannine who worked part time for us; she went through all their unopened mail and paid all their bills from all the un-cashed social security and pension checks; she made calls, wrote letters, and kept track of tedious details for these sisters. While the caregivers have been amazing, I think that Jeannine's efforts were what afforded these sisters the ability to live together, stay together, and keep all their finances in check. She has assisted in getting home repairs done, replacing appliances, and has been conscientious on every level to provide for these women for no other reason except genuine concern. Her devotion to these sisters is the biggest gift anyone could have given them.

Steve has also helped the sisters. Whenever Elsie needs anything, she calls Steve to order it from Amazon Prime, and if there is one mix-up with any order or item, she is back on the phone to Steve to get it fixed. He has also kept their home in good repair and made sure that the many maintenance and repair issues are handled. This is what a "care" company does when two humans have no one else but each other and can't do it themselves anymore.

One day in 2016, I got a call from our caregiver that Elsie was pale and weak. She could barely stand up. I told the caregiver that she needed to go to the hospital as this was a change in her baseline condition. Elsie was the more independent of the two sisters. Reluctantly, she left her sister behind and one of our caregivers met her in the ER and stayed with her so she was never alone. We also had to cover her sister, Mary Jo, at home with another caregiver as she has cognitive impairment and could not be left alone. The next day the doctor came in to tell Elsie she needed a blood transfusion. She refused the transfusion, and she called me. I went to see her and explained that the blood transfusion would help make her strong, and eventually, this would help her get home to Mary Jo faster. She agreed.

The next day they requested an abdominal CT scan, and Elsie refused. I sent Amy, our nurse, in to talk to her and explain why she needed it. She agreed to it. With each suggested procedure, Elsie needed some confirmation but was easily educated and agreeable. Her goal was really to get home to her sister so she recognized that being cooperative would help expedite that process, but she needed constant reassurance.

Since the CT scan showed tumors in her abdomen, Elsie needed a colonoscopy to find out where the tumors in her colon were located and exactly what type of surgery she would need, as it appeared that she definitely had cancer. Again, Elsie refused. I went over to the hospital to explain to Elsie why she needed the colonoscopy, and again, she agreed to it. Her colonoscopy was done on a Friday afternoon. She was given Propofol as a sedative—a very good sedative but one that makes your memory fuzzy for up to sixteen hours; hence, everyone is told not to drive a car and not to sign legal paperwork or anything else that could have legal ramifications over the course of twenty-four hours.

On Saturday morning, the doctor called me, as I was her medical power of attorney. He told me that Elsie had colon cancer and that typically he would recommend surgery for someone in this situation, but he was not sure he should do surgery on Elsie as she did not remember him post-colonoscopy. I reminded him that Propofol causes this type of amnesia and that this was not a good reason to not do surgery on Elsie. He initially told me that he was not sure that her life "was quality enough to save." At this point, I explained to him that Elsie had a very important role in life: to be there for her sister, Mary Jo, and while that may not be significant to him or to me, to Mary Jo it was her everything and her whole world. He reluctantly agreed to do the colon resection, and after explaining to Elsie that this was the final step before getting home, she agreed to it. When reminded of her sister, she was willing to do anything to be there for her—such devotion and love!

After the surgery, the anemia improved, Elsie went to a rehabilitation center and then, eventually, home to her sister. In a follow-up with the oncologist, Elsie expressed the desire to not have any chemotherapy, and the oncologist and I both agreed with her. We felt that having to take her out for treatments was not a good option, as this would be time away from Mary Jo and potentially life altering in a negative way in this circumstance.

Outcome :

It has been five years since her colon resection, and Elsie has never been sick a day since. She still sees her oncologist, who marvels at her success. These two sisters continue to live together, enjoy each day, and be with the most important people in each of their lives, each other. They still reside in their ranch-style home with 24/7 caregivers.

Mary Jo has slowly progressing dementia but knows she is at home with Elsie. She has a hearty appetite, is well cared for, and has a big smile on her face every day. Elsie has done extremely well, even to the point of talking about getting out and possibly driving again or doing some activities outside the home. Unfortunately, the COVID-19 pandemic has put the brakes on both of these agenda items, but there is joy in the Baker home, and I feel privileged to be a part of their life care plan.

Advocacy tips:

- Sometimes you have to fight/advocate for your patient to get all the procedures that the hospitalists and surgeons recommended. As the medical advocate for Elsie, I did what I felt was in her and her sister's best interest. Had the cancer been extensive and required much more in-depth treatment, like a colostomy or multiple organ resection, the conversation would have been much different.

- You need to be forthcoming with your patients. I explained to Elsie that any surgery has the risk of potential complications, including infection or even death. She understood this. I also told the doctor that I felt she understood the risks, and even if she did not make it off the table alive, we should do the operation since her sister's dependence upon her was worth the risk based upon their relationship.

· Chapter 15 ·

No Regrets

"Calmness is the cradle of power."

—J. G. Holland

After her husband died of a massive heart attack in his forties, Ann buried her husband and moved on, raising her seven children, ages seven to twenty-one. She got a job and remarkably became a wonderful provider for her children. She was a loving, nurturing mother who loved well. Her children had the utmost respect for her as she plowed through single parenting like a champ. In the blink of an eye, Ann went from a wife and mother of eight children to a single mother of eight.

Ann was a healthy woman who lived alone well into her nineties when she was diagnosed with a chronic lung condition known as bronchiectasis, where the lungs' airways become damaged, making it hard to clear mucus and increasing the chances of frequent pneumonia. She was becoming increasingly frail but was a private woman and did not prefer to have any help in her home. Her only daughter, Mary, was a big help to her, and began bringing meals once or twice daily to her home as she recognized that her mother was not eating as well and struggling to prepare food. Her mother was beginning to say that she was feeling as if things were changing but couldn't quite describe what that meant to her. Her family saw small changes in her gait, her ability to cook for herself stopped, and it soon became apparent that Ann was doing very little in her home each day. She was more fatigued and sat in her chair much of the day. Her daughter noted that she was not dressed when she arrived in the late mornings, like she used to be. Things were changing. Knowing that the time was coming for her mom to get some help, she reached out to me, but wanting to respect her mother's wishes, she wasn't forcing an in-home caregiver with her mother just yet. Then she got the call that Ann was on the floor and in pain.

Ann called one of her sons who came over to help and then they called 911. Ann needed to be evaluated for her injury.

The doctor found a small fracture in her femur and scheduled surgery. This was Ann's first surgery in her life! This fall would be the turning point for Ann's family, as they knew it substantiated the fact that Ann was weaker and needed more help. After a successful surgery with a pin in her femur and a small pneumonia due to her bronchiectasis which required antibiotics, Ann was on her way to rehab at a local facility.

She amazed her family over the next two weeks as she recovered and began physical therapy and even began walking, ten, twenty, and then sixty feet down the hall. For a while there, it looked like Ann was going to bounce back to her baseline. But around week three, fatigue set in, and Ann began to say, "I can't do this; please don't make me do this." As most children would do, they each tried to encourage her to push through, but she just did not have the energy to get through the day. She just wanted to be left alone; life was becoming a challenge for her. She even commented to her pregnant granddaughter, "I won't be here to see your baby." She just knew that her time on Earth was coming to a close.

I met with her six children on a Sunday afternoon to talk about moving forward with bringing help into her home. They all understood that Ann was fatigued and even doing physical therapy felt like climbing Mt. Everest to her. After several conversations with Ann, it was clear that she was ready for the end. We devised a plan to bring Ann home with hospice, allowing her the comfort and dignity of her own home. The physical therapist and the social worker agreed that Ann could no longer push herself, and she came home three days later.

Initially, Ann was not happy, but her sense of humor prevailed. She did not want a caregiver looking over her; it made her uncomfortable, so she thought maybe she should go back to the facility. But her family all rallied around her and helped her understand that they were all with her; the caregivers were just there to help them. She relented and became accepting, but stated over and over that she "wanted to go quickly." She would even joke from her bed, saying when she opened her eyes, "Am I still here? What time is it? If I wake up again and you're still standing there, I am going to be mad!" She had the family laughing at the bedside. She was ready to meet her maker, her family was on board, and she had a beautiful ending surrounded by her big, beautiful family five days later. Hospice provided wonderful services. Ann only had a caregiver for five days in her whole life, and her family was filled with satisfaction that she went just the way she wanted to go, quickly and with dignity.

Four months later, I called Mary specifically to see how she was doing with respect to her dear mother's passing: "I am doing very well. Of course, I miss my mother terribly, but I have no regrets." This is the feeling I want to have and that I wish every person could have after the death of a loved one. Ann had an arduous life on some level, but a beautiful, long life with an ending that she wrote for herself with her children executing the plan. This is quality of life, comfort, and dignity until the end. "No regrets" is what I want to hear and what I strive to hear with each and every patient that I work with. A sense of completion and peace that surpasses all understanding!

Outcome:

Just as Ann wanted, she got a quick and peaceful death surrounded by family. She was able to maintain her independence throughout her life and only had care for five days at home while in hospice, just as she desired. Ann was a strong woman who faced her death as she did her life: with humor and strength.

Advocacy tips:

Not all stories are like Ann's in that while many people do not want help in the home, it is truly imperative for safety reasons that someone is there to help them or to make alternative living arrangements. There are independent living communities (where no care is offered unless private help is hired, such as in Ann's case), group homes, assisted living facilities, skilled nursing facilities, and continuing care residential communities (CCRC) providing different living environments and levels of care throughout the aging process. There are for-profit facilities and non-profit facilities. There are Quaker, Jewish, and Catholic communities that offer aging in place and other religious-based housing facilities. There is a wide range. Decisions really don't need to be made until the safety of your loved one becomes an issue. This is hard for the patient themselves to see objectively, and it is at this point where families will often notice that their loved one looks tired or thin, or they are not following along with the conversations anymore and perhaps losing some of their cognitive ability. These are difficult conversations to have for any family.

· Chapter 16 ·

Return to Sender

"My whole life has been filled with joy through family, friends, neighbors and my nursing career."

—DLS, 2003

In early December 2018, Delores, whose medical journey was discussed earlier, went away with her big extended family to Deep Creek Lake for a pre-holiday getaway. Over forty family members gathered between two big houses to enjoy the weekend. This was a treasured weekend that no one would soon forget.

Delores had not been doing well prior to the trip, and over the course of the weekend, she continued to decline. She was short of breath, tired, and could not get comfortable no matter what she did. This was not a new issue, as she had had atrial fibrillation, COPD (chronic obstructive pulmonary disease), and CHF (congestive heart failure) for the past six years but managed to live without too many symptoms. Up until this weekend away with her family, Delores had managed to live alone in her home with part-time assistance. She needed help with bills, grocery shopping, and some light housekeeping, but she did all her own activities of daily living despite her legal blindness. However, the weakness, fatigue, and heart palpitations were becoming more and more of a daily concern leading up to this weekend. Then as the weekend progressed so did her symptoms, and it became clear on Sunday morning that she needed to be evaluated at a hospital. Her family opted to take her home and straight to her community hospital. On their way home, Delores verbalized that she was so grateful to have spent time with her family, and despite not feeling well, she would have opted to do it all again as time with family was what she described as "irreplaceable." She arrived in the ER and was triaged; within five minutes, she was whisked back to a room, and the rapid response team was paged to her bedside. Her heart was beating so quickly upon arrival that she was connected to monitors, on oxygen, and had labs drawn "STAT," a medical term meaning "immediately."

The rapid response team is the hospital's professional response team for individuals who are at high risk for heart attacks and strokes based on what the monitors are detecting. This is one step ahead of a "code blue" when a cardiac event has already occurred and an individual needs to be resuscitated. This team of professionals moves quickly and methodically usually to the bedside of the person in need within five minutes. The team includes physicians, nurse practitioners, physician assistants, nurses, lab technicians, and pulmonary specialists who swing into rapid action to save lives.

Atrial fibrillation causes fatigue related to the symptoms of an irregular heart rate, heart palpitations, and shortness of breath.

Delores's heart was beating at 150 beats per minute and unrelenting; she felt as if she was running nonstop on a treadmill.

After ten days at the hospital, she was sent to an acute rehabilitation center for two weeks. It was at this point in her life that she needed full-time round the clock private caregivers to help with all of her activities of daily living and personal care, but she was able to come home and celebrate the holidays with her family. Her family, grand-children, and great-grandchildren were very quick to come visit their grandmother for regular visits. She always provided positive encouragement to every person who came to see her and took an active interest in knowing how everyone's lives were going, and if there was anything that wasn't going well, she would support and share love with them.

She was thrilled to be in her own home, but at this point, her dose of Metoprolol was increased from 12.5mg per day to 200mg per day. This class of medication is called beta-blockers, and by slowing down the heart rate, they also tend to slow down one's entire system sometimes resulting in fatigue, depression, and overall sluggishness. This increase in dose made Delores feel almost completely vegetative. When I asked the cardiologist for another option, he did try some other medications, but Delores didn't tolerate them well and they did nothing to enhance her quality of life. She was feeling like a "wet washrag" with no energy and no spunk. Additionally, she developed a terrible rash from one of the medications, and the hospital cardiologist said we were out of options. She digressed from a completely independent elderly female to an almost vegetative state where even holding her head up was a chore. A-fib can do this in later stages; she had had this diagnosis for the past six years and had done well up until now with intermittent flare-ups. This was not only affecting her physical being but her mental capacities as well. She was being taxed to the point where it was hard for her to converse or stay awake for more than ten minutes at a time. With everything going on, she had many more bad days than what she would call "good days."

One weekend, she asked me to call the family together, as she truly did not feel she was going to live many more days. Dear friends gathered at her home and brought flowers and well wishes, and she even made some phone calls to classmates and relatives to tell them that she did not think "she had much more time on this Earth." One night she was staying at my home and asked me if I thought she was "ready" to leave this Earth. I told her that I felt she had lived her life in an exemplary manner and that if she had no regrets and it was her time, then I thought she could be ready, but I told her from my perspective there was "no hurry." We both laughed as I was powerless in this decision, and we both knew it, but I always marveled at how much she wanted to talk about this with me. While it was difficult to talk about, it was important to her and I wanted to honor her by helping her achieve "no regrets" as she approached end of life.

The next morning when she awoke, she recounted to me what had transpired during the night. She told me that she had gotten all the way to heaven and was standing at the doorway of a brightly lit opening but told "them" she wasn't quite ready to come in. She described in detail how the door closed, and she came back to her bed as it was obviously not her time. She calmly shared this with me and seemed fascinated by her journey, peacefully accepting that she still had a bit more time. She knew time was closing in on her, but again she wasn't afraid but remained more inquisitive and retrospective about her life.

She would continue to ask me if there was anything that could be done to help her current medical situation to optimize her quality of life. Feeling helpless as to what to do to help Delores, I opted to take her for another opinion.

What harm was there in trying an option to help improve her quality of life? She was asking for answers, which prompted me to seek out options. After the holidays were over, I took Delores for a second opinion to her original cardiologist who had not seen her in over six months due to the hospitalization and rehabilitation center stays that she went through. Delores looked much different than on previous visits, as she arrived in a wheelchair, head slumped forward, oxygen in tow, and barely able to mumble a few words. When her cardiologist looked at Delores and me, she said, "This is no way for her to live." Those were exactly my thoughts, as well as Delores's, but having been told there were no options, what choice did we have?

She explained that there was an option and, considering the poor quality of life that Delores was currently experiencing, she felt it would be worth the risk to pursue. She explained that twice in her career she had inserted a pacemaker in lieu of high doses of beta-blockers to control atrial fibrillation, and it changed the patients' lives. She explained that at ninety years old, the procedure came with risks, the most crucial one being death on the table during pacemaker insertion due to a myriad of potential complications. Delores herself said, "I feel like I'm almost dead now. I can't even hold my head up." Fatigue was 24/7, her mentation was sluggish at best, and the quality of her life had taken a nosedive since this last episode of prolonged atrial fibrillation and hospitalization. All along the journey, it seemed the evolving baseline became the "new normal."

With an elderly person, we can accept this reality to some degree, but if they have other options to improve quality of life, why not explore them? The family and Delores again discussed at length the quality of her life versus the quantity of her life. She had always been clear that she "loved life" but was finding this hard to accomplish with her current situation, especially given the declining cognitive function associated with her debility. We discussed at length with Dr. U if Delores could potentially regain her cognition. She told us it would take three months, but if she survived this procedure, her quality of life including cognition should increase greatly. She sounded very confident while disclosing all of the risks to us. She even told us that with a pacemaker, her CHF could also improve. This sounded too good to be true, but we went with it, and again, why wouldn't we?

Surgery was scheduled, the family was there for the send-off, a prayer was said at Delores's request, and off she went to the operating room with the family feeling hopeful, yet very vulnerable. What if this was the last time they saw her alive? They understood the risk but felt it was worth it to potentially improve her quality of life, as her day to day had become exhausting, draining, and hard to face.

The procedure went well, her pacemaker was set at eighty, and the electrical signals were ablated to allow the pacemaker to overrule the electrical signals and control the heartbeat at 80 instead of up to 150 beats per minute. Amazingly, over the next three months, Delores came back to her original baseline, which was happy, grateful, and conversant. She became more alert, lively, and gregarious. Her caregivers who started in December were amazed at her transformation. Even the heart rhythm specialist who performed the procedure could not believe the difference in this woman from when she was brought in on high doses of beta-blockers to now when she came in ambulating on her own and even asking the doctor how he was. He was shocked by her recovery and marveled at the cardiologist who made this call to "think outside the box and strive for a better quality of life."

Over the course of 2019, Delores's quality of life certainly improved, now off of the beta-blockers with improved cognition and a more normal daily routine. She got to go to her home in Pennsylvania in September 2019 for two weeks and thoroughly enjoyed visits from many friends and members of her extended family in her hometown. She was able to enjoy the weddings of two more grandchildren and many other family functions, her favorite pastime. She was able to attend a couple of garden club meetings and enjoy several visitors at her home.

The fall was smooth and steady for Delores. She enjoyed Thanksgiving and Christmas 2019 surrounded by family at her home. She enjoyed the noise, the fellowship, and the delicious food she loved to eat. Her life was joyous, and she was grateful for each day. We kept close tabs on her weight due to her cardiac issues (CHF) and fluid retention. By micro-managing her weight, we were able to adjust her medications and keep her symptoms at bay. When her weight increased and she retained fluid, her symptoms would get worse, and we would adjust her medications accordingly.

After New Year's 2020, Delores was steadily gaining weight related to her CHF, and no matter how we adjusted her diuretics or steroids, we were watching the needle on the scale creep upward. When we got to ten pounds above her baseline, I opted to take her to the ER for what I was hoping was a quick in and out for IV Lasix to pull some of the fluid off of her. She did get the IV Lasix that I was hoping for, and within four hours, Delores was back home.

Unfortunately, this did not do the trick, and her weight did not decrease as we had hoped. Her shortness of breath and exhaustion continued. We made a decision to go back to the hospital and realized that it would be a longer stay this time, as the in and out was not enough to therapeutically make a difference for Delores. So back to the ER we reluctantly went. When the physician asked me, "Do you know when she was born?" I knew we were starting off on the wrong foot. Of course, I knew what her date of birth was, but the bias of repeating her age intimated to me that we should have just stayed home and called hospice. Based on the past year and how well Delores had done, I did not think taking her to the hospital for diuresis was unreasonable. This hospitalization would prove to be what Delores called "my last time here (in the hospital)."

They did give her diuretics and Delores lost over ten pounds of fluid, which is what she came in for, but her new baseline was much more debilitated. While in the hospital, she was bedbound for five days and given a catheter so she didn't have to get up to go to the bathroom; consequently, she got weaker and weaker. One day when I was visiting Delores, I asked the nurse if she could please get up and go to the bathroom as it had been days since she had been on her feet, and her response was, "Oh, she can walk?" Her last day in the hospital started like this, and Delores's caregiver was with her around the clock when she was not accompanied by her family. Early in the morning, her doctor came in and listened to her lungs. Her caregiver Lia, out of concern said, "How do her lungs sound?" The doctor responded, "What do you want for ninety-five?" The caregiver texted me these words and was very upset by her interaction, as she felt that this was a very derogatory statement that was not accurate and did not answer the question that she was asking. She felt the lack of empathy coming from the physician, and she felt the age bias coming through. When the physician called me, I was ready for her call and prepared to tell her our plans.

The physician told me that Delores was not doing well at all and was continuing to decline; she now was diagnosed with worsening pulmonary hypertension on top of her CHF and atrial fibrillation. On top of that, the treatment seemed to be making Delores worse, as was the inactivity of lying in a hospital bed. She asked me what I thought should be the next step for Delores. Since the decline was obvious, I told her that the whole family wanted to bring her home and get her out of the hospital as soon as possible and coordinate hospice. The doctor felt this was a good plan as well.

That would be our last hospitalization "of choice" for Delores. We discussed this, and she told me that she did not want to go to a hospital again unless there was a situation that absolutely could not be handled at home. We had an amazing care team at home for her: our devoted nurse practitioner, Jessica, who helped me with medical decisions, our specialists who did curbside consults, and our devoted caregivers, Nellie and Lia. We could get almost any service we needed for Delores in the comfort of her home including labs, X-rays, and EKG studies. Comfort, safety, and quality of life continued for Delores, and I am grateful to this special woman who taught me so much about advocacy, nursing, and how to seek answers when appropriate.

Most importantly, this special person gave me the gift of life. Delores is my dear mother and has always been a person who loved life and spoke of her passion for living. She said that when her time came and her days were no longer quality, she was ready to return to her "sender." Because she believed she would ascend to a "better place," she wasn't afraid of dying. She knew that she was fortunate to have reached the age she was, and each night, she would express this gratitude to me, my siblings, and our offspring.

She knew she had been given many "bonus" years, as reflected in previous chapters, and loved the opportunity to have been able to watch her family grow and thrive.

Delores was my mother, my mentor, and my inspiration. She taught me how to love nursing by connecting with the patient and truly being present for every single person that we had the privilege of caring for. She truly felt that privilege was her mitzvah. Through her, I learned how to ask open-ended questions without being obnoxious or disrespectful, how to be passionate about good nursing care, and how to provide good follow-through care, and now I was able to return this gift to her by advocating for her life. She told me not to hold on to anger but to forgive and move on. Many times in my career as an advocate, I have fallen back on this advice. What a privilege this was for me: seeing her model how to enjoy the moments, even the rough times. She always took the time to find the silver lining and even had the courage to say, "If tonight is my last night, what an amazing life it has been." She showed me how to live life with no regrets and that a desperate situation still has its positives.

During the COVID-19 pandemic which started on March 16th, 2020, the entire country went into "lockdown." This meant we rarely left our houses for over three to four weeks until we felt a comfort level with even going to the grocery store. We wore masks and gloves and were told that this was an extremely contagious virus with a high fatality rate, especially among the elderly with multiple and pleasant words for them, and her face lit up during their exchanges. Never in our wildest dreams did we think that they would not get home for her final days, but that is exactly what happened. It was hard to believe but there were NO options to get them home safely. They knew they were deeply loved by their grandmother because she never missed an opportunity to tell them. Luckily, we were able to throw a wedding together in six weeks in 2019, as we knew Mom's condition was deteriorating and the bride-to-be told my son that she wanted to do this so his grandmother could be there. She was able to attend and actually "danced" at the wedding from her wheelchair. Their original plan was to be married in Colombia in July 2020, which was now canceled along with most weddings during the pandemic. Photos of the kids with their grandmother graced our homes and filled our hearts as we chose to focus on the gift we had been given versus the pain of separation at this difficult time. Mom also got to enjoy another wedding in 2019, that of her granddaughter Molly and husband, Will. She truly "lived" life to its fullest and did not miss anything. She would speak daily of her blessed life, beginning with her parents and one sister Corinne, who had five children that Delores was very close to. She very much loved my father, Jerry (fifty-two years of marriage), loved his family, and loved each of her five children who, in turn, gave her fifteen grandchildren, not to mention a son-in-law and four daughters-in-law. She imparted to us the importance of family and modeled unconditional love. She loved her neighbors and friends well, and as the quote states at the beginning of this chapter, truly lived her life with joy.

Two of her most frequent visitors were young neighbors, Noah and Will, who visited Mom regularly all the way from their toddler years to high school; she adored their visits and was truly interested in their lives. These boys had no idea the impact their visits had on my mother. She would actually well up with tears of gratitude as she remembered their visits over the years, especially their last visit in June when they came to the door in their COVID surgical masks to say "hello" before their vacation out west; Mom knew she would never see them again.

On July 6th, 2020, I set up an appointment for our primary care nurse practitioner to come out and evaluate Mom, as she continued to tell me that she was short of breath and began expressing fear. She would say, "I am scared, hold my hand." She even said this while we were already holding her hand or embracing her to reduce her fear. This "fear" was new and not an emotion common to my mother. After an honest conversation, we opted to bring hospice to the home. Because of the pandemic, I had held off bringing them, but it was time. Mom would tell me she was getting ready to leave this Earth but she "loved life, her family, and her friends." She told me how much she loved us children and our children and now her great-grand-children. She told us to honor her by continuing to care for one another and to never stop "sticking together." But more importantly, she modeled this. My son Chris counted forty-two calls between January and July 2020, and he was one of twenty-five family members that she would reach out to. Her red Jitterbug flip phone was her lifeline. She loved others well, she cared deeply, and she impacted change in many. She lived life to its fullest and taught us the same. Her positivity and optimism constantly echo in our minds and hearts.

Outcome:

In retrospect, the pandemic allowed us very special togetherness time with our mother. While others were so desperately lonely and many died alone, my mother was able to stay in her comfortable home with unlimited family visits. When I started my company in 2004, she asked me to please allow her to stay in her home "until she was taken out in a pine box." We were able to visit her, dine with her, laugh and cry with her. She had amazing care at home. We enjoyed many meals with her from all of her favorite restaurants. We would ask her what she felt like having for dinner, and then we would make it happen. We would give a shout out to the family, and whoever could make it would show up.

We knew her time was winding down. She would often ask me to sit beside her and talk about what "it" would look like for her. When she verbalized fear, we talked about it until she felt relieved of this feeling.

We would have conversations about her final days on a regular basis. While this was difficult, she wanted to talk about it. She was curious and expressive. We would laugh, and we would cry. She would tell me how much she was going to miss us, but I told her we would miss her more. I told her how grateful we were for her ninety-two years of love and life that she extended to so many. She even told me to tell the friends and neighbors that she could not meet with "thank you and goodbye."

She did manage the strength to call a few relatives and her dearest high school friend, Dotsy, to say goodbye. She was so brave and so grateful to each one she spoke to. Her favorite daily goodbye line to everyone was, "I love you big!"

In her final five months, she was able to meet the two newest members of the family: Her sixth great-grandchild, George Theo, was born in April and she was so excited to see whether Dara would have a boy or a girl. And in her last days, her seventh great-grandson was born five days before her last breath. Archer Van was placed in her arms just hours before she passed from this life. The circle of life was beautiful to witness, and she wrapped her arms around that child, unable to speak but still able to show her love. This will forever be etched in our memory, not a scene any of us will forget. Her sister's family all came to say goodbye on Sunday, and she passed on Monday. She knew everyone was there, and she enjoyed their visit. She literally ate and walked from her bed to her chair up until twenty-four hours before she passed. When Mom opted to no longer be hospitalized, it was OK with her family as they saw that each hospitalization took a toll. Quality of life was hers until the end.

Advocacy tips:

- End-of-life advocacy is easier if the patient wants to discuss it. Mom loved to talk about it and make sure she got to "check all the boxes."
- As an advocate, your end goal is comfort, safety, quality of life, and no regrets. Like Ann in chapter 15, we have been able to reflect with "no regrets." We miss our dear mother terribly.
- Sometimes it takes out-of-the-box thinking to allow for additional quality of life. We are grateful for the medical providers who tried different options and gave my mom more time.
- Always encourage your patient's families to use their village as support and always be mindful and return the favor when possible.

Just as she had promised when she knew I was writing this book, my mother indirectly sent me a title on September 12, 2020, by way of a returned letter she had written all the way back in September 2018 to my youngest son, Michael, who was supposed to receive it during his first week of college. The letter never got delivered to him but was returned in the mail to my mother with a "Return To Sender" label on it two months after she passed and two years after she sent it. Coincidentally, earlier that day, I had asked my mother (now in heaven) to please "show me a sign that all was well." Immediately, when I pulled the letter from her mailbox and saw the "RTS" on the outside of the envelope, the phrase "Return To Sender" resonated with me as the title my mother had promised she was going to send me.

The title is meaningful on many levels, as many of the gifts my mother shared with me were able to be "returned" to her in life and death. Her positivity and optimism will forever shape me and my nursing career. I continue to feel empowered by her gifts of mentorship in the field of nursing and the impact she left on my life. When I look in the rearview mirror, I can only see gratitude as I reflect on my parents' lives and what they gave to all of us. A huge shoutout to the entire Silbert crew, including Craig, Jessie, Saralyn, Evan, Holden, Tilghman, Alexandra, Molly, Will, Elin, Jeff, Wona, Taryn, Toby, Finlee, Maverick, Poppy Lorraine, Jantra, Tony, Luci, Archer, Dara, Steve, Joelle, George, Jarren, Randy, Landon, Mia, Steve, Matthew, Anamaria, Christopher, Michael, Curt, Lynn, Jonah, Brody, and Hudson—you all helped bless Mom's life with your love, visits, and time!

· Chapter 17 ·

Difficult Situations

"The measure of wisdom is how calm you are when facing any given situation."

–Naval Ravikant

This chapter contains information on how to deal with tough situations with a loved one or a dear friend. There is no script to follow. Each situation is unique and carries with it a different set of circumstances. While some of these issues are complex, there is always a solution and there are many more resources available than we know of when we are confronted with these scenarios. Don't be afraid to ask for help when you need it.

Share end-of-life plans with the entire family

My father died in 2003 at the age of seventy-eight. His death was not complicated. He had a forty-one-year history of diabetes, and he died of debility.

About three months before he died, my mother and I sat down and talked about my father's deteriorating condition with him and had a very frank open discussion after he commented that he was "tired" and did not want to start making hospital stays a part of his normal routine. He decided that he wanted his care to ensure comfort rather than to include corrective measures. Today that is the equivalent to palliative care, which helps people living with chronic serious illnesses and focuses on providing relief from the symptoms and stress of illness. The goal is comfort for the patient and their families. This seemed to be an easy solution that we readily agreed upon. But there was one problem. While my father, my mother, and I were all very clear on his decision, we made one huge mistake. We forgot to share this decision with the rest of my family, and one warm summer day, I was out running errands, and I got a call from my brother Jeff telling me that my father was having a difficult time breathing and he called 911. When they got to the house, my father was in cardiac arrest and my brother called me again to tell me this as they were about to start CPR. I told my brother, "No! No CPR! Dad had decided he doesn't want that, and we support his decision." But it was too late. As they were about to start CPR, my father's heart began to beat on its own. Due to the "differing of opinions of the family members," the 911 EMTs had no choice but to transport a patient such as this to the local hospital. Off Dad went to the ER. We raced to the ER and were met by a wonderful doctor who asked what our wishes were, and I explained the situation and he agreed to a "chemical code," which means oxygen, intravenous fluids, and medical support but no CPR or heroic measures. This was perfectly reasonable to the doctor as well as our family in conjunction with my father's wishes, and eight hours later, surrounded by family and a clergy member who had just prayed with my Jewish father, the clergy said "Amen," and my father took his last breath. No struggles, just a peaceful passing.

Takeaway: Advanced directives should be discussed and, in most cases, posted in the home to avoid confusion like this.

Be aware of a loved one's limitations

In 1993, I received a phone call from my parents' neighbor telling me that my father was OK but had been involved in an accident. When my father was backing out of his driveway to go to the store, his foot became stuck on the accelerator pedal of the car due to his peripheral neuropathy (a condition which impairs muscle movement and causes numbness in the feet), so he pressed the gas all the way down while in reverse, traveled over half a football field, and struck the neighbor's cement front porch and bounced his Buick's back bumper through the kitchen window. Fortunately, no one was home, but the structural damage was extensive and the house needed to be completely remodeled in the front with structural repairs. My father, while very shaken up, was not hurt. Again, while very grateful, we knew we needed to have some difficult conversations about this event. How could we allow him to drive knowing that this just happened and could happen again at any time?

This accident prompted major discussions around the table that evening. And we found out that my father had had "many near misses" prior to this incident. We told him that while it was just damage to a house and we were so grateful no one was injured, this felt like a warning call we needed to heed. If he could back out of his driveway at sixty plus miles per hour into a neighbor's home, what if this happened in a busy parking lot and people were standing nearby. He was shaken up enough to listen, and he never drove again after this incident. He willingly gave up the keys.

Takeaway: Discuss with your loved ones any health concerns you may have. My father never revealed to us his prior issues with driving. These concerns can cause embarrassment and lead to a vulnerability that many cannot handle. Subjectively these incidents appear very different to loved ones looking at them from a different lens. Yes, navigating your loved ones' difficulties with aging is not a perfect science, but we cannot control what we do not know, so it is important to be proactive and try to ensure they aren't hiding information.

When loved ones refuse help

I often see situations where adult children are at their wit's end about what to do with their parent(s) who refuses to accept their advice. I typically get the details of the situation and then weigh in when the safety of their parent(s) is at risk. I have had many meetings with adult children who feel their parents are at risk if they do not bring in help, but the parents refuse to listen, thinking the children are overreacting. Depending on the situation, I advise the children that if parents do not choose to be proactive in certain situations that are not dire, they can wait and see what happens. This is only an option if there is no emergent or dangerous situations going on at the time. If there is potential danger down the road, you can roll the dice and take the time to figure out what the best course of action is if the parents are not open to assistance. While this is not optimal, sometimes it is difficult if one parent remains competent and able to make decisions.

Once the parent(s) is at risk of harm to themselves or others, something needs to be done to protect them. There is a risk associated with stepping in when they have refused help, but most often their insight and judgement and reasoning skills are no longer intact, so what they see subjectively is quite skewed. I get at least one call a week regarding this very topic.

This situation happened with William, who was in the beginning stages of cognitive impairment but insisting that he didn't need help. "I can live by myself; I am perfectly capable," he used to tell his children. Since he kept insisting, the children continued to hesitantly agree that he could stay by himself. But in September, he was in his walk-in closet and somehow got locked in with no cell phone or means of communicating with the outside world for three days. His three children all lived out of state, and while they could not reach him, they did not raise any concern for three days until someone actually checked on him for a wellness check. There he was in his closet, hungry, thirsty, and in need of a good shower but not "injured" per se, except for the ramifications of dehydration and lack of nutrition for three days. He was hospitalized, and as hospitals will often do, the social worker indicated that the patient "was not safe to go home without oversight." This can mean that the loved one goes home with a family member who will provide this oversight, they go to a facility that will provide oversight, or they go home with caregivers who will provide this service. The hospitals are often the first to step in and dictate that a loved one can no longer live on their own safely.

If the patient refuses to have the oversight once they get home, they will actually send a caseworker out to the home and make sure someone is there, or they will send the patient back to the hospital and mandate that they get put into a facility.

Navigating situations where a loved one refuses help can be very difficult, especially if their spouse covers up for them, as they want to be the partner that helps in "sickness and in health." They want to protect their spouse and protect the children from worry or concern. Typically, I get a call before any major issue has occurred, but such issues are oftentimes right around the corner. It is usually about their loved one's memory failing along with their inability to remember to take their medications on time, or how to take them. It can be more serious like Mom took the car and was lost for hours and could not find her way back. Again, the spouse will try and rationalize why this occurred, like she didn't sleep well last night or she had a headache this morning. These little issues typically go on for a while before it is brought to the attention of the adult children. At this point, the children can then process this information in many different ways: they can minimize what they've heard, they can rationalize away what they have heard, they can step in and try to make big changes only to have them backfire, or they can put their parent's safety first and implement small, needed changes. Often

when the children identify an issue and request professional help for assistance in the home, the caregiver many
times will be turned away at the door. The loved one will
say, "Why is she here? I don't need help!" For this reason,
the children are so concerned that they will be accused of
not loving their parent or, worst-case scenario, be cut out
of any future gatherings or turned away forever. These
are fears adult children have, but concern for a loved one
who is having cognitive issues needs to be addressed,
especially when their safety may be compromised. It also
explains how a trip to the ER or hospital can help families
determine when an individual needs urgent intervention
as identified by the medical community and not the adult
children. It helps to have a neutral third party weigh in on
these difficult decisions to help prevent the children from
carrying all the burden.

Get advice on these difficult subjects to provide direction and professional guidance on the small, needed
changes you can make to ensure your parent's safety without changing so much that it backfires. Many wonderful
geriatric case managers and companies do this every day
and know exactly how to guide you. Unfortunately, aging
parents, especially those with cognitive impairment, lack
the insight and judgement to be able to understand subjectively what is happening in their life that is causing them
to be unsafe.

Because of this, there are resources, like APS, to help.
APS can intercede in urgent or dire situations to investi-

gate the safety and well-being of older adults. I have had to call them in on several cases in my career when I could not get a patient or their family to intercede in dangerous circumstances for whatever reason. APS is not adversarial and typically families will come back and thank me for getting them the help they needed. These situations are VERY DIFFICULT!!

Takeaway: When you face parents who do not want to listen to what you have to say, sometimes a third party is needed to listen to what you are seeing and make suggestions. There are more and more people utilizing LCSWs and RN case managers who can be very helpful in these situations.

When you can't be proactive, you need to be OK with being reactive. Aging is difficult for the individual as well as the family, especially if dangerous circumstances are emerging. Therapy can be very good for the adult children but not always feasible for someone with cognitive decline. Many unexpected challenges can surface, but fortunately, there are many resources available to help you.

Fear of upsetting your parents, or of losing their love and support are valid feelings, but if there is imminent danger, you must do the right thing to protect your loved ones.

When a loved one puts their vanity above their safety

Linda had repeated falls. I had worked with her spouse for several years, but now she was starting to have some balance issues. We discussed options including physical therapy and even using a cane or a walker. She told me "I would never be seen dead with a walker or rollator." Eventually, she fell right in front of her children at the mall and actually knocked her front teeth out. She spent several thousand dollars to fix them, and soon after that, she fell again. The second repair on her teeth made her stop and think. She was finally open to a change in her thought process, and we got her a rollator with the help of a physical therapist. After one week, she said to me, "Why didn't you make me do this earlier?" This actually increased her independence, as she can now safely exit the apartment building where she lives without the fear of falling. It has been several years now since she has fallen. She has so much more confidence and freedom, not to mention independence, back in her life. It is hard to impart wisdom, but eventually, we learn that vanity cannot replace safety.

Takeaway: Advice is not always heeded in a timely fashion. You cannot force change; you need to be patient and understand that your loved one is not ready, and in the interim, they may experience a fall or injury. While it is hard to accept, it is the way it is. Oftentimes, in retrospect, your loved one will do what Linda did and say, "Why did I wait to do this?"

When someone isn't capable of taking care of their loved one

One day I went to see one of my patients in her daughter's home for her first visit. It was not a clean house, and I had to step over lots of trash to get to the stairs, but I did not want to judge this patient's care by my initial impression of the home. When I ascended the stairs and entered the room of the patient, I found an elderly woman who would not speak to me. She looked terrified, but I was also a stranger so it was hard to know why this lady seemed so scared.

At that point, I began asking the daughter questions, and she seemed to be a caring, concerned daughter until I asked why her mother had a bruise under her eye. "I hit her," she told me. I asked her to repeat what she said, and again she stated, "I hit her. I had had a really bad day, and she was not cooperative, and I just hit her." I asked the daughter if she had told anyone besides me, and she said that she had told APS and they were working with her. I was completely appalled by her response and also somewhat skeptical of whether she had actually reported this incident. I called my boss as I left the house, since this was my first elder abuse case as an NP. We contacted APS, and they were aware of the situation and the daughter promised not to do it again. Unfortunately, two weeks later she did it again, and we were able to have the mother removed from this abusive home. The vulnerability of a nonverbal patient is multifaceted.

Takeaway: APS is a helpful agency. They look out for our vulnerable patients and will intercede when needed. Do not be afraid to contact them.

It's OK to change your mind

My friend Lisa's father, Mike, chose not to treat his invasive colon cancer after it was explained how extensive the surgery would be to remove part of his colon, his bladder, and his prostate. He was eighty years old at the time. Not only would he need a colostomy, but he would need a urostomy (procedure to allow urine to be collected outside the body) as well. He was so fearful of the complexity of this surgery that he opted to try chemotherapy and radiation and stop after that. When he finished his five weeks of chemotherapy and radiation, he was wiped out. He had mouth ulcers, no appetite, had lost forty pounds, and didn't recognize the skeleton in the mirror. It was hard, it was painful, it felt draining, and he was unsure he could go on. He was told by his doctors that this was normal after an arduous course of treatment like he had just been through and that he *would* get better; he just needed to be patient. Eventually, he started feeling better from this draining experience, just like his oncologist said. He began to eat, he slowly put on weight, and he threw himself a "celebration of life" party because he said he couldn't "make his own funeral" so he wanted to be alive to celebrate with his family and friends. It was an amazing party. Mike's plan was now to enjoy the life he had to the best of his ability, and when the time came, he would sign up for hospice services.

Then four months into feeling better, Mike had sudden abdominal pain, constipation, and vomiting; it sounded like an obstruction to me. Off to the ER he went, as the pain was unbearable. A scan was done and a large blockage from tumor growth was diagnosed. The doctor explained that the only option was surgery; the tumor had grown and was blocking his bowel. The man who never wanted a colostomy suddenly changed his mind. Maybe he could live with a colostomy? When facing the option of imminent death or a colostomy, the colostomy suddenly did not look so ominous. He chose surgery. He reversed his hospice mindset and instead opted for a colostomy bag. It was a hard adjustment for sure, and again, he was told to be patient. He did not want to look at it, touch it, or have anything to do with it. I told his daughter to support him and just give him time. Now nine months into it, Mike has adjusted to his colostomy, and he is glad he chose to do the surgery.

Takeaway: Mike is an inspiration to me and taught me to be open minded because it is OK to change your mind. He also taught me that one day I also want to throw a celebration of life while I am still alive and breathing. Thanks for the lessons, Mike! Hard decisions need support, and this family definitely provided support to their parents as they have both aged into their eighties, and they have adjusted their support as their parents' needs changed. Mike's daughter and my friend, Lisa, and her sisters have done a great job caring for both of their parents, adjusting to the constant turning tide of elderly parents and the challenges their illnesses present.

Ask for a copy of your labs or studies

Because you can get erroneous information, like what was conveyed to Delores in chapter 7, get a copy of your test results before you throw in the towel and give up. Remember the doctor recalled that Delores's CT scan in 2008 showed terminal bone cancer and was advised to "go home and get her affairs in order." Medical providers are busy people, and the best way to deal with a difficult situation is with the facts. I am at fault here too, because I did not question the results from the doctor. Fortunately, the radiology tech intervened and helped us figure out what was truly going on with Delores.

A similar situation happened with Roselle when she was told by her primary medical provider that her "blood work was fine." I asked twice for a copy and eventually was given a copy, which actually showed a significant anemia that required a blood transfusion. Do not be afraid to ask for important lab work and other medical studies when they are completed. They can be life savers.

Takeaway: Asking questions pays off. You don't want to harass anyone, but you want to have the facts. The same goes for emergency room visits and getting copies of all tests that were done. I feel like in recent years the hospitals have done a good job of sending patients home with their studies—blood work, X-rays, and scans—which is very helpful. Follow through is better when you have the facts in your hand and you aren't waiting for a fax or a phone call.

Helping loved ones with cognitive impairment

I work with a very well-respected geriatric psychiatrist who is adept at working with dementia patients with difficult behaviors. He has been making house calls to these underserved patients for fifteen years and is very good at understanding the disease and how to treat it. There are many neurologists, psychiatrists, and geriatricians who come in contact with these difficult-to-treat dementia patients and do not know where to turn. It takes a highly skilled medical practitioner to work with these patients and their families. Oftentimes, we will come into a home, and a family member will tell us that their loved one thinks it is December, and no matter what they tell them, they refuse to accept that it is, in fact, June and not December.

These arguments escalate and become very frustrating for both parties. I strongly urge all adult children or spouses to *not* engage in arguing with your loved one. It is pointless, it is shaming, and it gets you nowhere.

When we are with a family and an argument ensues, Dr. S tells the family, "It is more important to be kind than it is to be right." How true this statement is and how many families have benefitted from this statement.

There is no doubt that dealing with loved ones who have any type of cognitive decline is very difficult—perhaps one of the most difficult, as patients who have cognitive decline do not subjectively have any awareness of their decline and will challenge you on every single issue that is raised. They tell their family the same stories over and over, but the family members have to bite their tongues because admonishing them that they already told this story is shameful to them and makes them feel bad when they have no recollection of what they told their loved ones. On top of all the day-to-day struggles with cognitive impairment, they often won't accept help. If they will not allow you to bring in an advocate for them, such as a nurse, a geriatric case manager, or even their doctor, then you need to solicit help on your own.

Understanding dementia is frustrating for families of loved ones who suffer from it. Grasping a disease that is destroying your loved one's cognition, insight, independence, and life is difficult. Families need training or therapy with geriatric case managers or LCSWs to help them through this process. I have families that try everything they can to get their loved one to "accept or embrace" their diagnoses to no avail. It is irrational to think that an individual with cognitive impairment can rationalize and accept what is happening to them. Some turn to a therapist, thinking it will help their loved one understand, but it doesn't. Not even a professional can help them understand due to the patient's lack of memory and retention caused by their illness.

Takeaway: This is a very difficult medical journey to navigate. Caregivers need to step in and give families a break. Caregiver stress in a family member is real.

Remember to implement distraction with your cognitively impaired loved one; it may be the only way to break the cycle of their perseveration. Get them involved in exercise and socializing with kind, understanding people.

Remaining kind, patient and loving to your loved one with dementia is imperative. Do not shame them, bully them, or admonish them for something they have no control over. Many individuals with this disease were highly intelligent, productive members of society so treating them respectfully is a necessity.

If a loved one has dementia or any type of cognitive decline, education is the best tool for you. Sign up for a course or a support group and educate yourself. Accept that your loved one is not willfully trying to upset you with their repetition, but rather the disease is causing this behavior; they have NO control over it.

Implement a system that prompts your loved one to use the talents and abilities that they still possess. Encourage music, dancing, or art projects. We have artists that have continued to draw through their entire journey with dementia and we marvel at their masterpieces. Be kind to all patients no matter what their disease process is. They need your love and support, not your criticism and correction; it feels shameful and confusing to them and can contribute to their depression and frustration.

When they are done with their life

My patient, who was struggling with horrific hallucinations and chronic intractable back pain that could not be medically managed, told me several years ago that he "no longer want[ed] to eat. [He was] done with [his] life." The patient clearly told his family that his life was too arduous to continue at seventy-eight years old. He stopped eating and called his children to let them know. They all gathered around him to discuss his decision.

After listening to him, they all came to understand his very personal suffering and his lack of interest in taking multiple medications that did not seem to help. The process, of course, did not take long and hospice came on board within forty-eight hours to be a part of the care team. Ronald was made comfortable, his family stayed with him, and they laughed, cried, and shared with the time they did have. Once Ronald's life was over his family shared how special his last ten days were, and while they were deeply saddened by his death, they were comforted by his peaceful departure and that his desires were honored.

Takeaway: Sometimes it is just best to let your loved one go out on their own terms.

• Conclusion •

What's Next?

It has been a privilege to get in the trenches with some of these fascinating people and their families who all have amazing stories to tell about their lives and how they ended up where they are. Being there for others has become our passion and not just our business, which makes it such an interesting journey. Now you need to decide what is next for you.

For the advocate

We all have strengths and weaknesses that allow us to help others in specific ways. Not everyone is a born advocate.

Some people do not like discussing issues concerning health and medicine. Some people are too emotional to get involved in a loved one's health crises. But if you can handle it, you can become an advocate for a loved one in several ways.

- Meet with the patient themselves and discuss their situation
- Meet with the family members and see what their needs are as well as the patient's needs
- Connect people with the appropriate resources for their situation
- Research, educate, fact find, and seek out solutions to problems
- Get in touch with specialists, doctors, and treatment centers as needed for your patient
- Do not be afraid to seek out additional opinions from leading specialists in a given field
- Accompany patients on doctor visits, take detailed notes, and follow up as needed with physicians and patients to ensure goals are being reached

Use the tips given throughout this book to ensure successful advocacy, and good luck in your journey.

For the future patient

While you may be in perfect health right now, the time will come when you will face your own health crisis journey and may want an advocate. Many of us do not even contemplate our health or well-being until we are faced with an acute situation where we are forced to deal with the issue at hand. This is reactive advocacy. Some folks like to plan their living wills and have their advanced directives all written out; this is called proactive advocacy. While planning is optimal, not every situation allows for proactive advocacy.

When considering your future and who you want to have on your health care advocacy team, consider someone who is medical and maybe someone who also has legal skills; both careers interface with decision making and often arm an individual with the knowledge of how to pragmatically face an issue. Discuss your decisions with your chosen advocate(s) and make certain that they understand your wishes and concerns. The goals for my advocacy clients are the same through the continuum: safety, comfort, dignity, peace of mind, and quality of life. If you have different goals, express them to minimize disappointment. Allow a comprehensive assessment and update it as needed. Choose an advocate who will support your decisions wholeheartedly, not change directions at the last minute. My client Jeffrey (chapter 8) reviews with me on an annual basis what his desires are and, at this point, has even said he wants NO surgeries moving forward.

Unfinished business: Attempt to address any unfinished business from the beginning of your relationship with your advocate so as not to leave any stone unturned and, ultimately, to have "no regrets." The earlier these conversations are started, the less chance of missing the window of opportunity to discuss. Some of the important topics to discuss include who will take care of your family and what will happen with your home. I recently had a situation where a client passed away, and no one knew if she had a life insurance policy or how to track down her assets and liabilities. Find out about long term care policies that exist and don't be afraid to use them; a large percentage of people who have paid into a policy much of their life will want to "wait" to use this policy and often pass away without ever using the non-refundable benefit.

Desires/wishes: Discuss your desires, write down your desires, and if possible, draft them into a legal document, such as a Last Will and Testament as well as a Living Will and Medical/Legal Power of Attorney. Individuals who know that they do not desire interventions that prolong life should be as specific as possible when outlining their desires. This is helpful to know ahead of time. Identify your goals and communicate your plan. Meet with your advocate and show them where the documents are kept in case of emergency.

Confront your fears: What would bring you the greatest peace when confronted with end-of-life issues? State them, share them, and have them written down.

Meetings: Arrange to meet as often as you want. Meet up annually or at regular intervals to update your advocate on what you desire based on your life experiences that you have witnessed. Sometimes people will change their desires as life brings them more wisdom and challenges.

Gather your village: Bring family and community together in time of need; who is your "village"? Who gets notified if there is an emergency? The more your health issues are micromanaged, the more success you will meet on your journey. A goal-oriented focus helps keep your situation on track, but your advocate must have this level of comprehension to execute the plan.

"We cannot choose to have a life free of hurt. But we can choose to be free, to escape the past, no matter what befalls us, and to embrace the possible."

—Dr. Edith Eger

Thank you for taking the time to read my book about why I do the work I do. As Simon Sinek states, working hard for something we don't care about is stress, but working for something we love is called passion. Working with my clients is my passion. I love the challenges we face together on each journey. While I do not know all the answers, it is empowering to help every individual and family that I can. I have learned much from each and every person who has been placed in my path. Thank you for this privilege.

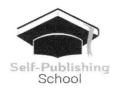

NOW IT'S YOUR TURN

Discover the EXACT 3-step blueprint you need to become a bestselling author in as little as 3 months.

Self-Publishing School helped me, and now I want them to help you with this FREE resource to begin outlining your book!

Even if you're busy, bad at writing, or don't know where to start, you CAN write a bestseller and build your best life.

With tools and experience across a variety of niches and professions, Self-Publishing School is the only resource you need to take your book to the finish line!

DON'T WAIT

Say "YES" to becoming a bestseller: **https://self-publishingschool.com/friend/.**

Follow the steps on the page to get a FREE resource to get started on your book and unlock a discount to get started with Self-Publishing School

ABOUT THE AUTHOR

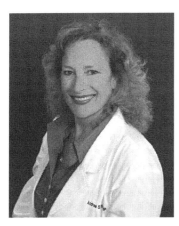

Andrea was born in Philadelphia, Pennsylvania and then moved with her family to Europe as a two-year-old. Living between France and Germany for four years helped shape her young life for adventure and world awareness. Being one of five children shaped her for nurturing and flexibility. From the age of six, she has resided in Montgomery County, Maryland. Being the daughter of a nurse and computer programmer and the only girl in the family led to many adventures, and competitive swimming was how she spent most weekends as she competed until her mid-thirties. She married a fellow she met in fifth grade, seventeen years after their initial meeting at Lakewood Elementary School. She graduated with a nursing degree from The Catholic University of America and later earned her Master of Science Nurse Practitioner degree at the University of Maryland in Baltimore. She started her own company in 2004, called Medical Consulting and Management, and was the last sibling to join the ranks of being an entrepreneur. Though a car accident right out of nursing school seemed like devastation for her career path, it actually helped shape and guide her into a nursing career that was far beyond her expectations. Making lemons into lemonade has always been her mantra and has brought her more satisfaction and contentment than she could have ever imagined. Add to the mix three active, adventurous, and amazing sons and now finally a daughter (in-law), life has truly never been boring.

In 2017, Andrea decided to give back on an international level and has been on three humanitarian missions. These exciting trips to Githunguchu, Kenya, Africa (near Nairobi); to Lesvos Island, Greece; to a Syrian refugee camp four miles from the Turkish border; and to Cambodia to help serve underserved humans in Kumar villages have fueled a passion within her. It is with complete gratitude that she looks in the rearview mirror and shares with you some of her journeys.

Made in the USA
Middletown, DE
20 June 2021